Workouts for Stepping into Emotionally Focused Therapy

Workouts for Stepping into Emotionally Focused Therapy is a companion to *Stepping into Emotionally Focused Therapy: Key Ingredients of Change* (2nd ed.). Inspired by Deliberate Practice, it is filled with exercises called workouts first with couples (EFCT), followed by a series of workouts in that same skill or move with individuals (EFIT).

The workouts are more than skill-drills. They are clear, tangible ways for the reader-practitioner to become emotionally engaged within self and in attunement with each client scenario and to strengthen their EFT muscles with the practice of each of these EFT ingredients of change. Part 1 includes workouts of ten micro-skills across a wide range of client scenarios, including diversity of racial, ethnic, gender, sexual orientation, religious, neurodiversity, and other contextual diversity. Workouts with the five moves of the EFT Tango, from beginning of therapy to the completion of Stage 2 change, first with a couple and then with an individual, make up Part 2. The reader-practitioner has opportunity in Part 3 to apply the macro-intervention to Stages 1 and 2 change in their own lives, to explore barriers to following and deepening emotions, and to utilize a series of antidotes for typical EFT therapist challenges and goal-setting.

Containing practical handles for the new clinician or graduate student wanting to integrate EFT into their practice, it is also stimulating and relevant for seasoned therapists and counselors seeking to sharpen EFT skills and develop confidence in the model with both couples and individuals.

Lorrie L. Brubacher, MEd, Director of the Carolina Center for EFT, adjunct at UNCG, Greensboro, NC, has authored many EFT training videos, articles, and chapters. She trains in EFT internationally.

"*Workouts for Stepping into Emotionally Focused Therapy: Exercises to Strengthen Your Practice* is **the** guide for clinicians practicing EFT. Brubacher is a gifted writer who beautifully details the most relevant micro and macro skills while prioritizing culture and context. Each workout broadens and builds, bringing EFT to life in the reader's own words. A remarkably unique resource for every EFT therapist!"

> **Kathryn Rheem**, Ed.D., LMFT, EFT Trainer, Co-founder of the EFT Café, Co-director of WBCEFT, co-author of *The Emotionally Focused Therapy Workbook for Relationship Loss: Healing Heartbreak Session by Session*

"In this excellent new book, Brubacher provides Micro-Skill Workouts for mastering key skills in EFT. The text is clear, well-organized, accessible, and highly effective. Very highly recommended for both EFT trainees and certified therapists who wish to take their EFCT and EFIT skills to a new level!"

> **Dr. Tony Rousmaniere**, Program Director, Sentio University Marriage and Family Therapy Program, author/editor of Essentials of Deliberate Practice APA Book Series, President-elect, Division 29 of the American Psychological Association (Society for the Advancement of Psychotherapy)

"In *Workouts for Stepping into EFT*, Lorrie Brubacher helps therapists, from apprentices to the most experienced, learn all the nuances of applying EFT to both individual and couple therapy. With her gentle guidance, the reader is invited to focus on the core micro and macro interventions of EFT. As they further develop their understanding of each intervention's purpose, they can practice applying it and draw inspiration from Emily – a fictive therapist – to help them expand their repertoire, discover and solidify their strengths, and integrate the model conceptually and experientially – so they can find their own voice as EFT therapists. This book is a must-have for anyone wanting to master the art of EFT."

> **Dr. Caroline Gasparetto**, Certified EFT Therapist and Supervisor, Co-founder of EFT Québec – collective winners of the ICEEFT North American John Douglas Award for 2023, for significant contributions to the growth of EFT, Lecturer at Université de Sherbrooke, Co-founder of EFT and Me, a webinar series

Workouts for Stepping into Emotionally Focused Therapy

Exercises to Strengthen Your Practice

Lorrie L. Brubacher

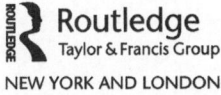
Routledge
Taylor & Francis Group

NEW YORK AND LONDON

Designed cover image: Photodisc © Getty Images

First published 2025
by Routledge
605 Third Avenue, New York, NY 10158

and by Routledge
4 Park Square, Milton Park, Abingdon, Oxon, OX14 4RN

Routledge is an imprint of the Taylor & Francis Group, an informa business

© 2025 Lorrie L. Brubacher

The right of Lorrie L. Brubacher to be identified as author of this work has been asserted in accordance with sections 77 and 78 of the Copyright, Designs and Patents Act 1988.

Library of Congress Cataloging-in-Publication Data
Names: Brubacher, Lorrie L., author.
Title: Workouts for stepping into emotionally focused therapy: Exercises to strengthen your practice / Lorrie L. Brubacher.
Description: New York, NY: Routledge, 2024. |
Identifiers: LCCN 2024020553 (print) | LCCN 2024020554 (ebook) | ISBN 9781032151328 (hardback) | ISBN 9781032151311 (paperback) | ISBN 9781003242666 (ebook)
Subjects: LCSH: Emotionally focused therapy. | Couples therapy. | Family psychotherapy. | Psychotherapy.
Classification: LCC RC489.F62 B783 2024 (print) | LCC RC489.F62 (ebook) |
DDC 616.89/1562—dc23/eng/20240509
LC record available at https://lccn.loc.gov/2024020553
LC ebook record available at https://lccn.loc.gov/2024020554

ISBN: 978-1-032-15132-8 (hbk)
ISBN: 978-1-032-15131-1 (pbk)
ISBN: 978-1-003-24266-6 (ebk)

DOI: 10.4324/9781003242666

Typeset in Times New Roman
by codeMantra

Support Material

Additional material, including chapter summaries and exercises, can be accessed online. Please go to www.routledge.com/9781032151311 and click on the link that says Support Material. A link to the supplementary material will appear.

For Alison Claire Lee 1946-2023
Friend and Colleague
EFT Trainer and Supervisor Extraordinaire
Your light, your love, your laughter, your leadership shine brightly over the
entire EFT world!

Embodying the heart of humanistic therapy, you said,
"Our clients are good people who have simply lost their way."

Fostering creativity, confidence and capacity in every supervisee and trainee
to integrate the core of EFT with their personal style, you said,
"Everyone will sprinkle EFT with their own Pixie dust."

Teaching and modeling the core of emotionally focused therapy and
the complexity of the process of emotion, you said,
"Every emotion has a story!"

May this book, in some small way, help to keep your loving spirit and your
EFT light burning brightly in new and seasoned EFT therapists, across the
globe, who never had the opportunity to meet you in person.

Contents

List of Workouts

Additional micro-skill workouts are in Part 1 Support Material available at routledge.com/9781032151311

Book Description

Workouts for Stepping into Emotionally Focused Therapy is a companion to *Stepping into Emotionally Focused Therapy: Key Ingredients of Change* (2nd ed.). Inspired by Deliberate Practice, it is filled with repeated exercises called *workouts* first with couples (EFCT), followed by a series of workouts in that same skill or move with individuals (EFIT).

The workouts are more than skill-drills. They are clear, tangible ways for the reader-practitioner to become emotionally engaged within self and in attunement with each client scenario and to strengthen their EFT muscles while practicing key EFT ingredients of change.

Part 1 includes workouts of ten micro-skills across a wide range of client scenarios, including diversity of racial, ethnic, gender, sexual orientation, religious, neurodiversity, and other contextual diversity. Workouts with the five moves of the EFT Tango, from the beginning of therapy to the completion of Stage 2 change, first with a couple and then with an individual, make up Part 2. The reader-practitioner has an opportunity in Part 3 to apply the macro-intervention to Stages 1 and 2 change in their own lives, to explore barriers to following and deepening emotions, and to utilize a series of antidotes for typical EFT therapist challenges and goal-setting.

About the Author

Lorrie Brubacher, MEd, LMFT, RMFT is the Founding Director of the Carolina Center for EFT. Certified with the International Centre for Excellence in EFT (ICEEFT) as a therapist, supervisor, and trainer, she has worked in private practice in individual, couple, and family therapy since 1989, and has private practices in North Carolina, USA, and Manitoba, Canada. She has an adjunct appointment at UNC Greensboro and has previously been an instructor at the University of Manitoba, University of British Columbia, and University of Winnipeg. She publishes and presents internationally on EFT, having taught Emotionally Focused Couple Therapy (EFCT) and Emotionally Focused Individual Therapy (EFIT) since 2009. Lorrie has co-authored six chapters with Dr. Sue Johnson, the originator of EFT, a chapter with Dr. Ting Liu on online EFT, and is published in the *Encyclopedia of Couple and Family Therapy,* in the *Journal of Marriage and Family Therapy,* in *Person Centered and Experiential Psychotherapies*, and with Dr. Stephanie Wiebe on Process Research to Practice in the *Journal of Family Psychotherapy*. She serves on the editorial board for the international *EFT Community News* and is a contributing author to *Becoming an Emotionally Focused Therapist: The Workbook* (2022). She is co-developer, with Dr. Lillian Buchanan (2014) of the first EFT interactive video training program, AIRM, accessible at www.attachmentinjuryrepair.com and has many EFCT and EFIT training videos available at https://steppingintoeft.com/. She has written this book as a companion to *Stepping into Emotionally Focused Therapy: Key Ingredients of Change* (2nd ed.) with the first edition (2018) available in nine languages, with more translations in progress. See more at www.lbrubacher.com, www.carolinaeft.com, and www.eftandme.com.

Foreword

S. M. Johnson

Workouts for Stepping into EFT is an excellent companion to Brubacher's main text, *Stepping into Emotionally Focused Therapy: Key Ingredients of Change* (2nd ed.). Used together, these books are sure to strengthen competence, confidence, and joy as an EFT therapist. Both books shine with simple, down-to-earth language that is straight-forward and practical for therapists wanting to strengthen their practice of EFT.

Creating the model of EFT, initially for couples, and expanded to work with individuals and families, has been a labor of love for me. I am thrilled to see many colleagues, the world over, continuing to foster the growth in EFT with the same passion and enthusiasm I have had for creating and expanding this integrated experiential, systemic model, rooted in the revolutionary science of attachment theory. Brubacher's *Workouts for Stepping into EFT* is an accessible resource for therapists seeking a boost of encouragement and concrete ways to integrate this evidence-based model of EFT into their work with couples and individuals.

This is the first book with applied exercises with both couples and individuals throughout each chapter. This integration is sure to enhance therapists' understanding of the EFT model and EFT Tango across modalities, thereby increasing their capacity to put it into practice. It provides therapists with an opportunity to grow in both the art and science of EFT because of the unique nature of each practice exercise (called a *workout*). Prompts and guidelines to attune to one's inner somatic experience and cognitive processes while also attuning to clients, and forming each micro-skill or EFT Tango move, immerse practitioners in rich experiential learning. The theory and rationale for the workouts are made clear, yet there is plenty of room for artistry and diversity in how the therapist responds. This book compels practitioners to taste what it means to attune to clients and to seek a felt sense of clients' experience in their own bodies, before forming any interventions in response. The workouts are solidly attachment-based, bringing the supremacy of attunement and the power of emotion alive in very vivid and concrete ways. Workouts also prompt therapists to attune to both attachment threats as well as contextual threats, consonant with the new focus on sensitivity to racial, ethnic, and cultural sensitivity in Brubacher's second edition of *Stepping into EFT*.

Readers of the main text will already be familiar with Emily, the fictitious therapist learning to practice EFT. She is present in this book as well, providing her best attempts to respond to the workouts after the reader creates their own response. Her sample responses are gentle examples for the reader to compare with theirs, without conveying there is one correct answer for any of the workouts in the book.

The progression of the book is focused and relevant: The first section focuses on deliberate practice of ten micro-skills, providing engaging workouts, that are sure to strengthen all your

EFT muscles and to help you discover EFT muscles you didn't know you had. The repetition of each micro-skill with multiple client scenarios illustrates the richness of the simplest of skills. The workouts provide much more than repeated skill drills, however, because each one is based on the internal and interpersonal experience of the therapist with the couple or individual client. This provides an opportunity to develop and solidify your own EFT language and style as you practice the exercises. Having ongoing feedback from "Emily" as to her responses encourages practitioners to appreciate diversity of responses and to name their strengths and growing edges. Certainly, as Lorrie suggests, the benefit of each workout will be enhanced if done with one or more colleagues. The value of exploring a diversity of styles from different colleagues and receiving encouragement for one's own capacities cannot be overstated.

The second section of the book applies the EFT macro-intervention – five moves of the EFT Tango to two extended cases – one EFCT and one EFIT. Multiple workouts are engaged through a course of Stages 1 and 2 change events. This section is very different from the micro-skills workouts earlier, in that there is a cumulative buildup where one workout leads to the next, in an interconnected web of supporting client change through the model, with the moves of the EFT Tango. Therapists are helped to see there is more than one way to respond. They are encouraged to experiment with the very specific intentions of each of the EFT Tango moves, rather than being provided with the "correct answer." Although Emily's responses are provided for most workouts, the reader is continually reminded that it is ok if their response is different from Emily's, but that the important thing is that they are experimenting with the specific goals of that particular Tango move.

Finally, the third section is related to the self of the therapist. As Brubacher suggests in the introduction, it may be a good idea to simultaneously work through some of Part 3 alongside the client scenarios in Sections 1 and 2 of the book. Part 3 is a great way to experience the power of the EFT model for one's own stuck patterns and struggles. The section on antidotes to common EFT therapist struggles also fits well with the goal-setting practitioners are encouraged to do throughout the book.

The book itself is grounded in attachment theory, in that it provides a secure base and a safe haven for therapists seeking to learn and grow in EFT. It focuses on helping the practitioner validate their EFT strengths in every workout. Each workout ends with an invitation to reflect on personal strengths or things the practitioner likes about the intervention they have just formed, as well as to identify what they may wish to add to their style from the example response given by Emily. The workouts are designed to hold your hand with very practical, theoretically congruent prompts and to build on the reader-practitioner's strengths. Psychotherapy is a challenging task and it is also a practice of love and hope. Human transformation and growth is a most exciting and humbling process in which to participate. This practical book is sure to enhance your competence in the empirically validated interventions and the attuned artistry that are bedrocks of EFT.

S. M. Johnson

Preface

Workouts for Stepping into Emotionally Focused Therapy (EFT) is a practical companion to the text *Stepping into Emotionally Focused Therapy: Key Ingredients of Change* (2nd ed.), Routledge. The *workouts* are intended to be an exciting discovery tool that appeals to a range of therapists, from those enthused about deepening their competence in EFT, to those struggling to find confidence and proficiency as an EFT therapist. You may find yourself at different places on that continuum, depending on the client challenges you are facing on a particular day. Becoming an EFT therapist is an ongoing journey of personal and professional development over time, commonly filled with thrilling periods of enthusiasm, mixed with some discouragement, confusion, and self-doubts. The *workouts* are structured to provide a gradual yet focused and validating experience of stepping into a new paradigm. As with therapist identity development in general, there can be periods of demoralization (Watkins, 2012) and fluctuations between feelings of mastery and chaos (Skovholt, 2012). The good news about embracing the journey to become an EFT therapist is that therapists report a more empathic, collaborative stance toward themselves as therapists and toward clients following EFT trainings (Conrad, 2015; Koren, Woolley et al., 2022; Rodríguez-González et al., 2020; Sandberg & Knestel, 2011).

In the world of athletics, *workouts* are a period of physical exercise to improve fitness, ability, or performance. Musicians, executives, athletes, and most recently, psychotherapists, with the many collaborative endeavors of Rousmaniere (2019) and colleagues (Rousmaniere et al., 2017), apply deliberate, repetitive practice to develop skill and excellence in their specialty.

Requests from readers of the first edition of *Stepping into EFT*, as well as from online trainees from across the globe have motivated me to write this companion workbook. Specifically, requests from colleagues for concrete, practical EFIT and EFCT applications have helped to create my vision for this exercise book.

The term *EFT workouts* was initially introduced together with my EFT trainer-colleague, Ali Barbosa, in 2018 when we began offering training sessions named *EFIT Workouts*. *Workouts* for increasing fitness and competency in the practice of EFT with individuals were introduced as a metaphor for the primary goal of EFT – to shape *emotional fitness* – the flexibility, connectedness, and resilience that come with reprocessing emotional experiences through interpersonal, emotional dialogue. From an EFT perspective, client goals, while collaboratively shaped and expressed in ways that mirror the specific client's circumstances, are variations on the interconnected themes of *emotional flexibility and attachment security*.

Workouts in EFT, by virtue of the need for the therapist to be emotionally engaged, are necessarily more than drills in specific skills. They are emotionally engaged exercises, compelling therapists to engage in emotional attunement before formulating words with which to respond and then to reflect on their responses. Each *workout* is accompanied by a sample response from Emily, the therapist featured in the companion book, *Stepping into EFT*. Prompts are given for the therapist to compare their responses and to identify their strengths and anything new they wish to integrate into their style of being an EFT therapist.

The *workouts* will be enhanced if they are done together with one to three colleagues. My ongoing experience is that trainees are encouraged by their experiences in *workout* practices when they share and learn from each other. It is a marvelous way to build confidence and to be enriched by discovering different ways of doing EFT.

Naming the book and the exercises *EFT Workouts* is also to convey a playful nature to what can be a steep learning curve of becoming an EFT therapist. It is hoped that therapists engaging in these *workouts* can find some pleasure, like venturing out on a summer scavenger hunt, encountering an array of challenging client scenarios and stuck points, with clear directions for how to follow emotion and attachment through the mazes of case formulation and shaping change events.

The EFT *workouts* are exercises designed to evoke readers' participation and engagement in applying EFT interventions throughout the model with different client cases, and to facilitate therapists' reflection on their own processes when engaging with various couples and individuals in distress. Commensurate with *deliberate practice* (Rousmaniere et al., 2017) the *workouts* provide incremental practice of the attunement, micro-skills, and moves needed to undertake the three main EFT tasks – building alliance, deepening emotional experiencing, and shaping corrective emotional experience through affiliative interactions in order to facilitate the EFT stages of client change (Brubacher & Wiebe, 2019; Greenman & Johnson, 2013; Johnson, 2019).

Emily, a fictional, white, cisgender, heterosexual female therapist, introduced in the main text, *Stepping into Emotionally Focused Therapy: Key Ingredients of Change* is also present in *Workouts for Stepping into EFT*. She is earnestly seeking to broaden and deepen her EFT skills and be racially and culturally sensitive in doing so. During many online EFT trainings, she was thrilled to discover colleagues from around the globe with varied socio-cultural contexts, all seeking to learn EFT! She treasured her interactions with colleagues, engaging in the search for how to enhance competence and flexibility by applying EFT across modalities of couple and individual therapy. The universal relevance and applicability of the EFT model across varied cultures and different contexts continue to impress her. At the same time, she is discovering how the EFT interventions are precisely adaptable to particular nuances and distinctions for different cultural contexts and cultural expectations. The *EFT workouts* in this book are created for EFT therapists like Emily and colleagues from across cultures to help them fine-tune their EFT practice. Emily's responses to the *workouts* are also given. Therapists are encouraged to team up to support one another in their learning adventures by inviting one or more colleagues from different contexts to engage with them in deliberate practice of the *EFT workouts*.

Acknowledgments

Alison Lee, Co-founder of the International Centre for Excellence in Emotionally Focused Therapy was the fuel and the light that empowered me to write the first edition of *Stepping into Emotionally Focused Couple Therapy: Key Ingredients of Change* (2018). Her inspiration and belief in me sustained me through the second edition of that book and this companion exercise book. I hope this book helps to infuse many therapists and clients worldwide, with her loving, validating, brilliant, agentic EFT spirit. Thank you for your friendship, your intellect, your laughter, and simply for all of who you are!

In addition, I want to acknowledge several very special friends and colleagues who gave me the encouragement to keep on with this book when the road seemed too long. To Ali Barbosa, Mexico, Dimitrij Samoilow, Norway, and Jackie Evans, Ottawa, Canada, for reading drafts and seeing the potential in my plan, thank you! Also, Ali and Dimitrij, thank you for supporting me in birthing the initial *workouts* in groups with you. Thank you to Feion Villodas for sharing your expertise and yourself, patiently and kindly, challenging my attempts at racial and contextual humility, and for being an ever-available resource. I learned much from you and have much more to learn! Your influence permeates this book. In particular, thank you to Caroline Gasparetto, Montreal, Canada, for lighting a torch in the last seven months and encouraging me, *workout by workout*, with her diligent reading and responding. Thank you for all your tireless encouragement! Without your almost daily inspiration and cheerleading, I cannot imagine I could have seen the way through these final laps!

To Sue Johnson, first and last, thank you for believing in me and supporting my endeavors! Thank you for inviting me to write the first edition *of Stepping into Emotionally Focused Couple Therapy*, which in turn gave birth to a second edition and to this companion book of EFT *workouts*.

Thank you to all my friends and family, especially Shannon and Josh, for still being there when I have been absent for far too long. Finally, gratitude and love to my endless encourager who tolerates and celebrates me every day, my dear husband, Dan Perlman. Thank you for listening and listening and listening, and always being cheerful and full of good ideas and love.

Introduction

Attachment theory, like many spiritual teachings guides us to restore the dignity of relationships and to find effective emotion regulation through relationships. Emotionally Focused Therapy (EFT) works to help people move from patterns of emotional distress and isolation to *broaden-and-build* cycles (Mikulincer & Shaver, 2023) of emotional fitness and interconnection. EFT asks and answers – How do we create secure bonds? How do we create *shalom* as in the Hebrew scriptures – living in harmony with each other? How do we foster a sense of connection to a larger whole the way New Zealand Māori regard their *whakapapa*, their genealogy, as a place of sacred belonging? How do we work in our isolated therapy offices with an attachment-based model built on community? Many therapists are drawn to EFT because it is built on interconnection and on the power of emotion as the target and agent of change in attachment relationships. At the same time, we need to honor our limitations to sense another's racial, cultural, and contextual experiences that differ from our own experience. We need to slow down with humility and curiosity to notice verbal and non-verbal *emotional* and *cultural handles* that can open doors to a richer experience of a client's world.

Strengthen EFT Muscles to Follow Signals of Emotion and Attachment

Written as a companion to *Stepping into Emotionally Focused Therapy: Key Ingredients of Change* (2nd ed.), *Workouts for Stepping into Emotionally Focused Therapy* (EFT) is an engaging, practical application of following the attachment map toward change through EFT. EFT is an empirically validated model of psychotherapy relevant across modalities of couple, individual, and family therapy. In *Stepping into Emotionally Focused Therapy*, the reader meets Emily, a young therapist keenly invested in learning EFT and expanding her skills, particularly in the modalities of Emotionally Focused Couple Therapy (EFCT) and Emotionally Focused Individual Therapy (EFIT). EFFT examples are outside the scope of this book, though engaging in these *workouts* is sure to fine-tune your EFT muscles across all modalities of individuals, couples, and families!

Engaging in the EFT *workouts* compels a therapist to first, enter their inner process of attuning to one client or one interpersonal dynamic at a time; second, to formulate a micro-skill or an EFT Tango move in response to the client; and third, to compare their intervention to Emily's, thereby identifying their own strengths and specifying new facets they wish to integrate.

Workouts in Part 1 are designed to give you repeated opportunities to practice ten EFT micro-skills that are used in the EFT macro-intervention, the EFT Tango, first with couples (EFCT) and then with individuals (EFIT). Following *workouts* in ten micro-skills, Part 2 provides you with opportunities to integrate these micro-interventions into the five moves of the EFT Tango – the EFT macro-intervention. Johnson's metaphorical reference to the macro-intervention of EFT as a series of five (tango) moves originates in her discovery, as an Argentine tango dancer, that the five moves of the tango resemble the deeply connected attunement and improvisation of an attuned EFT therapist. Two case examples introduce the moves of the EFT Tango, through the course of therapy, first with a couple in EFCT and second, with an individual in EFIT. Then, *workouts* to deliberately practice attuning and responding with repetitions of the five specific moves of the EFT Tango are given, first with a couple and then with an individual, through the stages of EFT change. Personal reflection exercises are interspersed throughout all the *workouts* to guide therapists to focus on attunement to client and to self, while deliberately formulating the EFT micro-skills and facilitating client change with the moves of the EFT Tango.

Congruent with the *bottom-up* (experiential) nature of EFT, developed from observing how clients change, Part 3 provides exercises to bring the model to life for you personally. Entitled "The Self of the Therapist," this section guides therapists to experience the benefits of the EFT change process for themselves as they engage on the receiving end of the EFT micro-skills and moves. Personal reflection and journaling exercises direct you through Stage 1 and Stage 2, to experience the EFT change process for yourself. You can extend these personal workouts with a peer – exchanging roles as discloser and engaged responder – after your own self-reflective journal writing.

Common challenges faced by EFT therapists are delineated, accompanied by EFT antidote resources to these challenges. The reader is encouraged to identify their specific strengths and to set one or two goals at a time for continued growth. The antidotes to common challenges faced by EFT therapists and suggested guides for your own professional goal-setting provided in Part 3 will be helpful ways to monitor your own development as you do the workouts of Parts 1 and 2.

If you have already read *Stepping into EFT: Key Ingredients of Change* or another introduction to EFT and are familiar with the model, you may find it helpful to take a look at Part 3 and to switch back and forth between the earlier parts and Part 3, as you make your way through the main *workouts* in Parts 1 and 2. Part 3 is designed to specifically nurture and support the person of the therapist and you may find taking forays into Part 3 to be a refreshing way to nourish yourself as you do the *workouts*, and to continue setting new goals for growth and celebrating your progress.

Unique Features

This book is unique in the field of therapy workbooks and exercise manuals in four ways. First, for each practice exercise (called a *workout*) you, the reader, are given guidelines of inner somatic and cognitive processes that a therapist can follow to form each micro-intervention and therapist move. Prompts for focusing your inner processes and attunement, while forming interventions help to demystify what may seem like magic or pure artistry and intuition to novice EFT therapists. Guidelines to focus your awareness on specific facets of your inner process and attunement before formulating your response help you apply the science and artistry of a skilled EFT therapist.

Second, after being guided to insert your responses in writing, you are provided with Emily's inner processes in forming her responses and then you are offered the response that Emily makes. You are reminded that Emily's is *not the one correct answer*; it is Emily's response and you are then invited to reflect on how your responses are similar or different from hers and to identify your strengths and discoveries of anything new you may want to add or integrate into your style of being an EFT therapist.

Third, *working out* alongside Emily, a fellow companion on your EFT journey, gives you an opportunity to grow stronger together. In this way, it is hoped you will also see the value of doing these exercises together with a colleague, thereby discovering different styles of executing the same interventions and principles and building one another's strengths and a spirit of collaborative encouragement.

Finally, the couple (EFCT) workouts followed immediately by individual (EFIT) workouts, give practical evidence that EFT is one attachment-based model. Couple and individual applications are different modalities of the same model. There are many similarities and yet some specific nuanced differences (Johnson, 2019). The actual workouts provide ample evidence of two key similarities between EFCT and EFIT. First, attachment theory informs therapeutic interventions and offers a de-pathologizing, growth-orientated clinical basis for case formulation of human misery and motivation to change. Second, restructuring emotional experience as it occurs in session is at the core of a model that shapes change through interpersonal dialogues, known as in-session *encounters*.

You are encouraged to extend the workouts to your personal case examples. Recording and reviewing therapy sessions is how to learn EFT. We learn from our clients and from observing how accurately we are attuning and facilitating the processes of reflecting, assembling, deepening, shaping corrective emotional experiences through engaged encounters, and processing and integrating these experiences. While reviewing your therapy videos, you are encouraged to excerpt one or several client statement(s). Then, following the prompts for a specific micro-skill or move of the EFT Tango, given throughout the book, formulate your response, and reflect on your strengths and growing edges. The prompts for formulating each EFT micro-skill and EFT Tango move are given with such simplicity and detail that it is hoped you will insert your own clients' expressions and create your own specifically relevant workouts to practice between sessions.

The workouts also highlight some nuanced differences between EFCT and EFIT. In EFCT, the couple dyad in the room is the focus for stabilizing patterns, restructuring the bond, and consolidating change across the partners' lives, whereas in EFIT the focus is the individual's typical pattern for regulating emotion – an active internal/interpersonal process across relationships with significant others who populate their inner world. With couples, the key therapeutic focus is helping partners to restructure their attachment bond into one of security and this has the impact of shifting working models of self and other. EFCT has been shown to effectively reduce individual symptoms of depression and post-trauma reactions. With individuals in therapy, on the other hand, the focus is on restructuring strategies for engaging with life where effective co-regulation replaces depression, anxiety, and post-trauma reactions. For example, in Part 2.3, Samir's depression and post-trauma reactions reveal unexplored grief and relational injury. Reprocessing this grief and emotional pain, a clear voice of assertive anger, meaningful connections, and confidence emerge.

In both couple and individual modalities, the focus extends beyond symptom reduction to building trusting bonds and meaningful enthusiasm for being fully alive. Interpersonal connection leads to stronger and more resilient selves, capable of effective dependency. Optimal dependence on others leads to resilient autonomy and continuing personal and relational expansion.

The clinical examples in the workouts have been inspired by real clients. Some excerpts are similar, but not identical, to what you will find in training videos available at steppingintoeft.com or in the scenarios in the companion text, *Stepping into Emotionally Focused Therapy*. Other workouts are composite case examples, created for the workouts.

Most workouts contain: (1) Some context and a client expression; (2) Prompts for you to insert your inner process and attunement; (3) Space to insert your EFT micro-skill or EFT Tango move; (4) Samples of Emily's inner process and attunement; (5) Emily's micro-skill or EFT Tango move; and (6) Space to insert your thoughts about your strengths and discoveries about what you want to add to your practice, when you compare your responses to Emily's.

The time you take in each workout to reflect on your inner process will be longer than you have in real life. You are invited to take time to engage with your inner experience and self of the therapist's presence in these micro-steps of forming interventions to fine tune your attunement skills and to enhance your proficiency in the EFT micro-skills. The one series of *workouts* where you are not given time to reflect on your inner process before you jump right in to respond are the *catching-the-bullet workouts* in response to aggression expressed toward a partner in the room or toward self in EFIT. This is because of the urgent nature of this micro-skill where interruption and immediate audible reflection of the present process is how a therapist grounds themselves to move close to clients with a combined reframe-conjecture to regain safety.

Emotion

Emotion is the agent and target of change in experiential and attachment-based psychotherapies. "*Emotional agility*" (David, 2016) also heralded outside the world of psychotherapy, is a touchstone and a byproduct of relational and mental health. "In EFT, health is described as the ability to fully listen to and engage inner experience (particularly emotional experience), to trust this experience, and to create meanings that can then direct behavioral responses" (Johnson, 2009, p. 411).

Micro-Skills and Five Basic Moves

EFT micro-skills comprise the five basic therapist moves that Johnson (2019, 2020) refers to as the five moves of the EFT Tango. **EFT Tango Move 1** (reflecting present process) is important for building and maintaining the therapeutic alliance (safety/understanding) and for engaging with the present moment throughout therapy; **EFT Tango Move 2** (assembling and deepening emotion) is needed for creating coherence and validation and deepening emotional experiencing); **EFT Tango Moves 3 and 4** are needed for shaping corrective emotional experiences through affiliative interactions, known in EFT as engaged *encounters*; finally, **EFT Tango Move 5** is needed for summarizing, integrating, and consolidating change

The EFT macro-intervention, the EFT Tango, is not a new model. It is the same model described in Johnson (2004, 2019, 2020) and in Brubacher (2018) and *Stepping into EFT* (2nd ed.). Therapist processes and interventions, described in the deceptively simple, yet very rich EFT Tango metaphor, however, are taking center stage in current EFT training and some current literature. The stages and steps of the empirically validated model do remain as a guiding map of where clients are and where they need to go. (See Chapters 13 and 14, in *Stepping into EFT* for details on markers of client steps and stages and Tables 1.1 and 1.2 for specific steps and stages in EFT. Throughout that companion text, EFCT and EFIT details and examples are provided.) The *workouts* are focused on therapist interventions with some references to how the micro-skills and tango moves are used differently across client steps and stages of change. The five moves of the EFT macro-intervention guide EFT therapists, as process consultants, to attune and collaborate with clients and to help them move through the EFT stages of client change – from the four steps of assessment and de-escalation/stabilization, through the three steps of restructuring attachment processes, and finally to the two steps of consolidation and integration of the corrective emotional experiences into pragmatic changes across relationships and contexts of a client's life.

Steps and Stages of Client Change Very Much Alive in the Background

There are specific EFT steps and stages of change that clients take on their pathway to health, optimal dependence, and attachment security. In these EFT *workouts*, therapist processes and interventions take center stage, while the EFT map of client steps and stages of change moves to the background. This is commensurate with the discovery by Johnson and colleagues that many therapists new to learning EFT were finding a predominant focus on the steps of client change to be too complex as an initial guide for practicing EFT. Focusing on the macro-intervention of the five basic moves of EFT has been found to engage therapists more effectively in helping clients move through the EFT change process. Readers are given *workouts* to incrementally practice the EFT micro-skills and EFT Tango moves that they can then use to walk with clients through their steps and stages of change.

As mentioned, the stages and steps of client change, outlined in the companion book *Stepping into EFT,* remain a very important map to locate where clients are and what steps they still need to take to reach their goal. The map of client change indicates the route the clients take. The same therapist interventions are used across all steps and stages of client change, however, as seen in the Tango *workouts* in Part 2, are tailored to where clients are on the map of change.

In Stage 1, the micro-skills and moves are used to help clients form a solid alliance with the therapist, identify the problematic pattern maintaining their distress, and access the core underlying emotions and unmet attachment needs driving the pattern. By helping clients to own their strategies for engagement, new meanings and action impulses arise and clients are able to reframe their distress as their automatic pattern of reactivity and self-protection given their unmet longings.

In Stage 2 restructuring, the EFT micro-skills and moves, especially Moves 2–4, are used in a slower, deeper, more deliberate way to deepen and disclose more vulnerable emotional experience and to structure clear reaches and responses for attachment needs. Client emotional flexibility increases and secure attachment bonds are formed. As newly positive patterns of reaching for, responding, and receiving emotional support are initiated, views of self and other shift. Views of self as lovable, competent, and worthy emerge; views of other are discriminated to clearly see those who are dependable, accessible, and responsive. Moves 1 and 5 are also used in a more intense way to track and integrate the corrective emotional experiences shaped in Stage 2.

Clients' new strategies of emotionally congruent reaching and responding are the *broaden-and-build* cycles of attachment security (Mikulincer & Shaver, 2023) that are consolidated in Stage 3 of EFT, across various problems and life contexts. During consolidation, the same EFT micro-skills and moves are used, but in a less intense way with more of a focus on summarizing and integrating the changes created throughout therapy.

Therapist Interventions

The *workouts* provide therapists with opportunities to increase their own awareness and skill development in applying the science and the art of EFT (Johnson & Brubacher, 2016). The *workouts* are a series of repetitive practices in therapist micro-skills and moves. The interventions are oriented to the key clinical implications of attachment science – the three main tasks of EFT: First, forming and maintaining a therapeutic alliance; second, harnessing the power of emotion; and third, shaping emotional dialogues to create emotional flexibility, fitness, and new working models of self as worthy, lovable, and competent and distinguishing key others who are reliably accessible and supportive.

Therapist Awareness of Presence and Interventions

An EFT therapist needs awareness of both how they are utilizing/experiencing their presence in relationship with the client and how they're using EFT interventions to maximize the power of emotion and interpersonal dialogue to clear the path for the client to move toward their optimal destination of effective dependency. My intent with these *workouts* is for you to practice, practice, practice the EFT moves and micro-skills – and to reflect on your inner experiencing while doing so. Emily and colleagues remind each other, "As process consultants, EFT therapists are not attempting to *change clients*. Rather we are attempting to *join with them* in a collaborative process of helping them to create corrective emotional experiences – interpersonal dialogues that create lasting shifts." The *workouts* are oriented to help EFT therapists enhance their capacity to be aware of self as an active experiencer and responder in dialogue with clients, thereby becoming better positioned to attune, to bring emotional experience to life, and to help clients reprocess their experience moment-to-moment to create *broaden-and-build* patterns of secure bonds and effective emotion regulation.

Additional micro-skill workouts can be found in the online support material at routledge.com/9781032151311.

Part 1
EFT Micro-Skill Workouts

The following set of workouts offers you practice in ten EFT micro-skills. In order to become skilled in the EFT macro-intervention, the EFT Tango, a therapist needs to be familiar with the micro-skills that make up the five moves of the EFT Tango. These attuned moves are used across every session to help clients step through the stages of the EFT change process.

Each micro-skill is introduced, followed, first by EFCT workouts and secondly, by EFIT workouts in that same micro-skill. Each workout contains context, a client expression, prompts for you to insert your inner process and attunement; prompts to form your particular micro-skill response; Emily's inner process and attunement, and her version of the particular micro-skill response. You are invited to compare your responses with Emily's, not as a check for correctness, but to identify strengths in your unique style of EFT and to make a note of anything you see in Emily's response that you may want to integrate into your EFT *way of being*. Detailed directions, given in the first workout for each micro-skill, are to be followed for each subsequent workout in that micro-skill. Although the prompts are not given each time, you are encouraged to read each client's expression and your and Emily's responses aloud, to experience the full impact of the words and to get a felt sense, each time. Various clients reappear across workouts.

We begin with empathic attunement, which is the imperative inner process that a therapist needs to formulate each micro-skill. You are encouraged to return to workouts in attunement at any point, because increasing your conscious awareness of your empathic attunement will enhance your capacity to practice each of the micro-skills. Following this are workouts in empathic reflection, evocative responding, validation, and heightening. These are staple micro-interventions needed to work with EFT as an integration of experiential, systemic, attachment-based, and culturally-humble therapy. There is a brief set of workouts on therapist transparency or self-disclosure. After this are workouts in more complex, micro-skills, including empathic conjectures (reflections on the *leading edge* of what clients have shared) and reframing (the backbone of this de-pathologizing model of therapy that sees the problem residing not in a person, but in rigid, repetitive patterns of insecure attachment strategies and interactions) and several micro-skills that combine conjectures and reframes, known as *seeding attachment* and *catching bullets*. The final workouts on catching bullets include three workouts on repairing ruptures in the face of therapist faux pas and micro-aggressions.

Some micro-skills require more practice than others and you will have opportunities to continue practicing them in concert with others as you move through the EFT Tango workouts in Part 2. An online supplement includes additional micro-skill workouts (see routledge.com/9781032151311). Several additional EFT micro-skills included in Part 2 are tracking reflections, refocusing/

DOI: 10.4324/9781003242666-1

redirecting, summarizing, and a special type of conjecture, known as *slicing it thinner*, used while shaping encounters.

The micro-skill workouts are designed so that you can use them in applications with your own clients. The prompts to guide your own inner process and attunement and the prompts for how to form each micro-skill can be applied to any client expression from your sessions as you review your videos or check your notes. If you are feeling stuck with a particular client, couple or individual, follow the prompts of each micro-skill to attune to a challenging client more deeply and then formulate a micro-skill that can move the process forward. Follow the workouts to strengthen your EFT muscles with your own client examples. Have fun and enjoy the journey!

EMPATHIC ATTUNEMENT TO THE CLIENT'S PRESENT-MOMENT EXPERIENCE

Attunement requires the therapist's active engagement, walking around in a client's world as much as they can, employing their *empathic imagination* to get a felt sense of the client's experience. Before an EFT therapist formulates any words to reflect what they hear and see, they taste and feel in their own body the verbal and non-verbal messages from the client. They slow down to honor their limitations to sense another's contextual experience. Slowing down helps the therapist to notice verbal and non-verbal *emotional* and *cultural handles* that can open doorways to a richer experience of a client's world.

Attunement is a fundamental part of formulating all EFT micro-interventions, yet it is easily overlooked. If we as therapists slow down enough to consciously notice the rapid, limbic process of attuning, we multiply exponentially the profound resource of the person of the therapist and the resonance between clients and therapist. Being aware of one's attunement helps therapists to be more fully present, to enter more fully into their clients' worlds, to monitor and repair the alliance, to track emotions as they come alive, and to create and maintain safety while shaping and processing encounters. Attunement is needed for every micro-skill in the EFT Tango.

How to Attune to Client's Present-Moment Experience

1. Identify an emotional handle (verbal or non-verbal) that strikes you as the most poignant part of the client's message.
2. Observe your reactions while attuning to the most poignant part of the client's message: your body, thoughts, feelings, and impulses to action.
3. Notice if your reactions pull you close to the client or their partner or pull you away from the client or their partner.
4. Curbing your readiness to assume you *fully* understand, identify an item of empathic curiosity that you have that could help you to enter more fully into the client's world.

Note: This set of workouts is all about your felt sense of attunement as you resonate with your clients. Thus, you do not need to create a verbal response. After each client expression, you are given prompts and space to record your inner attunement. You then have an opportunity to read Emily's response. This is not to tell you how you *should* attune, but rather to give you an example of one therapist's attunement. First, reflect upon your own authentic attunement and then read about Emily's attunement. Next, take the opportunity to compare your responses with Emily's and to make some notes of what you like about your attunement and empathic curiosity and any discoveries you are making about how you could sharpen your own empathic attunement and curiosity prior to formulating any words to the client.

EFCT Empathic Attunement Workouts

EFCT Empathic Attunement Workout 1: Ping-li and Roger in Desperation

Context A heterosexual couple, Ping-li and Roger in an early session. A more pursuing partner, Ping-li is complaining that her quiet and withdrawn partner, Roger, is unresponsive.

Client Expression
Read the client's expression in this and each of the following workouts below aloud as though you were the client(s). Then follow the prompts to insert your inner process and attunement.

PING-LI: I'm just so frustrated – drained, foggy, tired. I just have to take care of myself – just like Roger is doing. (Voice heightens, almost to a whine.) He will never return a favor for me, that is becoming more and more clear, so I am just in survival mode. (Voice drops.) He said he's looking after himself. (Falters; voice becomes more fragile – like walking on eggs.) And I need to too!

Your Inner Process and Attunement

1. Identify an emotional handle (verbal phrase or image or non-verbal signal) that strikes you as the most poignant part of the client's message: _____
2. Resonate with this emotional handle and observe your internal reactions (in your own body, thoughts, feelings, and impulses to action). What are they? _____
_____
3. Do your reactions pull you close to the client or her partner or pull you away from the client or her partner? _____
4. Curbing your readiness to assume you *fully* understand, identify empathic curiosity that could help you to enter more fully into client's world: _____

After inserting your authentic attunement responses, compare your responses to Emily's below and see if you discover any ways to deepen your own attunement and empathic curiosity without the pressure to formulate any words to the client. Your attunement may be similar to or very different from Emily's responses. The goal is to deepen your awareness of your emotional felt sense (inner bodily, cognitive, affective, relational, and curiosity).

Emily's Inner Process and Attunement

1. Emotional handles Emily identifies: fragile voice saying, "in survival mode; take care of myself."
2. Emily's internal resonance: As she resonates with this emotional handle, she has the following reactions.

<u>Body</u> – bracing tension initially, then opening and softening in chest; tension for Roger who is listening to accusations and complaints about him.

<u>Thoughts</u> – how do I contain this escalation and support this fragility without alienating her partner, Roger? Stay calm. Join with both partners. She hears a very frightened Ping-li in survival mode, frightened and alone.

<u>Feelings</u> – compassion, eagerness, and slightly frightened.

<u>Impulses to action</u> – Interrupt to reflect and contain. Initially, she feels annoyed with Ping-li's whining. As Ping-li's voice becomes fragile and her face drops Emily feels herself pulled in to want to offer comfort.

3. Pulled close to or away from? After an initial pull-way feeling Emily feels drawn toward Ping-li's desperation and fragility. She also feels drawn to what she imagines is a precarious position for her partner, Roger, as he is being blamed and possibly misunderstood.

4. Curbing her readiness to presume understanding, Emily imagines Ping-li's accusations of Roger may have a larger context that she doesn't yet understand. She is curious to learn more about what triggers Ping-li's sense of needing to take care of herself and about what "survival mode" means for her.

Your Strengths and Discoveries about Empathic Attunement

After comparing your response with Emily's, make some notes of what you like about your attunement and empathic curiosity and any discoveries you are making about how you could sharpen your own empathic attunement and curiosity prior to formulating any words to the client.

_____

_____

_____

EFCT Empathic Attunement Workout 2: Ping-li and Roger, Falsely Accused

Context

Roger, Ping-li's partner from the above workout, reacts to what he hears as accusations that he doesn't look out for his wife and that in her eyes he is unreliable.

Client Expression

ROGER: (After Ping-li accuses him of never looking out for her, only for himself, and of being very undependable.) Wait! (Voice loud and excited; head jolts back, look of surprise.) That's unfair! I'm falsely accused! I haven't made any plans to leave! She does make me happy! She *is* enough!

Your Inner Process and Attunement

1. Emotional handle: _____

2. Your internal resonance (body, thoughts, and feelings): _____

_____

3. Do your reactions pull you close or pull you away from Roger? _____

4. Area of empathic curiosity to help you to enter more fully into the client's world: _____

_____

Emily's Inner Process and Attunement

1. Emotional handle: Emily identifies as an emotional handle, Roger's most poignant message, excitedly saying, "Falsely accused! This is unfair…she does make me happy!"
2. Emily's resonance: As she resonates with this emotional handle, she has the following reactions (body, thoughts, feelings, and impulses to action).
    <u>Body:</u> Emily feels tense and hot in her body and slightly unsteady about containing two partners in self-protection mode, starting to escalate.
    <u>Meanings:</u> She imagines that Roger must have felt accused of looking out only for himself and is now pushing against Ping-li, while also seemingly in a panic that she is pulling away to take care of herself. The urgency she hears in his voice seems as though he is almost pleading with her not to give up.
3. Pulled close or pushed away? Emily's first impulse (her action tendency) is more of a pull away – wanting to explain to the partners what they are doing. Becoming aware of her explanatory pull-back mode, Emily shifts to wanting to move close to understand more about how triggered Roger seems by what Ping-li has just said. She is also curious to find out how Roger's reaction is impacting Ping-li.
4. Curbing her readiness to assume understanding and find empathic curiosity to enter more fully into Roger's world, Emily curbs her readiness to assume he is panicking or defending himself and becomes empathically curious to learn more about his excitement and surprise and what it means for him when he says, "This is unfair…she does make me happy!"

Your Strengths and Discoveries about **Empathic Attunement** and curiosity prior to formulating any words to the client. _____

_____

_____

EFCT Empathic Attunement Workout 3: Jack and Karen, Stabilizing Yet Struggling

Context
Jack and Karen are stabilizing. They both say that things are so much better than when they began therapy, which was at the time that Karen discovered Jack texting with other women.

Client Expressions

JACK: We've definitely made progress. We weren't getting along and weren't communicating. It was just the whole *fussin' and cussin'* and just making it worse. It was like we were going in circles when we talked. The same things just kept happening and happening and happening over and over. All the time we would say, "Let's just talk about it," but nothing would get solved. It would stay the same, but we are definitely making progress now.

KAREN: I agree. We are listening to each other much more than before. But I think sometimes it's maybe why we bicker a little bit more is because he's finally voicing his opinion, whereas he didn't used to. So, we butt heads. I mean, we get through it, but we have so much going on in our lives. We are both struggling a lot and we still bicker too much.

Your Inner Process and Attunement

1. Emotional handle: _____
2. Your internal resonance (body, thoughts, feelings): _____
_____
3. Do your reactions pull you close or pull you away from Jack? _____
4. Area of empathic curiosity to help you to enter more fully into the client's world: _____
_____

Emily's Inner Process and Attunement

1. Emotional handles:
   Jack: We were going in circles; making progress now;
   Karen: both struggling and still bickering too much!
2. Emily's internal resonance:
   <u>Body</u>: Emily feels a slight spinning in her chest.
   <u>Meaning</u>: Jack is positive, yet Karen seems troubled; confused about what to feel – senses hope from Jack and discontent from Karen.
3. <u>Emily's action tendency</u>: Drawn to Jack; hesitant toward Karen.
4. Curiosity: Curbing her tendency to assume Jack is "trying to look at the bright side" and ignore their distress, she is curious to hear more from Jack about what "progress" means for him and curious to hear more from Karen about how she sees them "each struggling."

Your Strengths and Discoveries about **Empathic Attunement** and curiosity prior to formulating any words to the client. _____
_____

_____

See the online supplement (routledge.com/9781032151311) for more EFCT empathic attunement workouts.

EFIT Empathic Attunement Workouts

As was noted at the beginning of the EFCT empathic attunement workouts, this set of workouts is all about your felt sense attunement as you resonate with your clients' present-moment experience. Thus, you do not need to create a verbal response. After each client expression, you are given prompts and space to record responses about your inner attunement. You then have an opportunity to read Emily's response. This is not to tell you how you *should* attune, but rather to give you an example of one therapist's attunement. First, reflect upon your own authentic attunement and then read about Emily's attunement. Next, take the opportunity to compare your responses with Emily's and to make some notes of what you like about your attunement and empathic curiosity and any discoveries you are making about how you could sharpen your own empathic attunement and curiosity prior to formulating any words to the client.

EFIT Empathic Attunement Workout 1: Ivy, Substance Use and Losses

Context

Ivy describes herself as caught in cycles of using substances and being sober. She has survived the death of her partner by suicide and the recent death of her beloved dog. She is currently sober, participates in 12-step groups, and is a 12-step sponsor for others. She is a psychiatric social worker.

Client Expression

IVY: I've just got to get on … just be an adult. There's no point in fretting over my losses or my guilt. (Pause.) I lost my partner to suicide. (Pause.) No one loved me like she did. (Pause.) But I don't blame myself for that. I lost my job because of using drugs. Can't feel sorry for me. That was my doing! I lost my sweet dog but he was really sick. Couldn't save him, though I tried! He was my baby!

Your Inner Process and Attunement

1. Emotional handle: _____
2. Your internal resonance (body, thoughts, feelings): _____
_____
3. Do your reactions pull you close or pull you away from Ivy? _____
4. Area of empathic curiosity to help you to enter more fully into the client's world: _____
_____

Emily's Inner Process and Attunement

1. <u>Emotional handle:</u> Emily identifies a resounding sense of loss, even as Ivy speaks dismissively and nonchalantly about her losses. Ivy's words about her partner, "No one loved me like she did" and "I don't blame myself for her suicide" strike Emily as especially poignant.
2. <u>Resonance:</u> As she resonates with this emotional handle of loss, she has the following reactions (body, thoughts, feelings, impulses to action).
   Body – Emily's heart expands.
   Meanings – Ivy has had so many losses – especially losing the one person who loved her more than anyone; there are many things she says she does not feel – no guilt, not sorry for self.
   Feelings – Emily feels protective toward the client, and compassion for her many losses.
   Impulses to action – Emily wants to slow Ivy down, and help her notice what she is saying.
3. Emily feels drawn to the client. She feels compassion for her losses and her scattered pace that doesn't seem to allow her to notice her own experience.
4. Curiosity: Curbing her readiness to assume she can fully understand, she identifies that she wants to discover more about Ivy's experiences of loss; to learn more about her experience of losing the person who loved her more than anyone else. Also, she is curious about what "not feeling guilt" and "not feeling sorry for self" mean for the client. (See note on p. 13.)

Your Strengths and Discoveries about Empathic Attuning

_____

_____

EFIT Empathic Attunement 2: Joy, Exhausted But Moving On

Context

Joy identifies as Christian and African American. She routinely gives emotional and financial support to her family, including her mother, her sister, and her nephew. She works in middle management in a rapidly growing business, receiving increasing demands from her supervisor, while at the same time finding that those, she is supervising, are needing increasing amounts of support. She is struggling with exhaustion, but as she says, "The way we are raised as African Americans is to just move on and not attend to how difficult things may be."

Client Expression

JOY: (In a matter-of-fact tone, like reporting facts.) I cannot step back … even though I am exhausted. I would be leaving my mom alone to deal with everything on her own. Knowing that she feels like I'm the only person that she can confide in, not wanting to be a disappointment. I cannot let my staff down. They could lose opportunities for promotion. No, I cannot step back. Not anywhere. But I don't let things get me down. As a Christian, I am taught to sacrifice for others daily and as an African American, I must just keep going.

Your Inner Process and Attunement

1. Emotional handle: _____
2. Your internal resonance (body, thoughts, and feelings): _____
_____
3. Do your reactions pull you close or pull you away from Joy? _____
4. Area of empathic curiosity to help you to enter more fully into the client's world: _____
_____

Emily's Inner Process and Attunement

1. Emotional Handle: Emily identifies the following emotional handles: Exhausted but cannot let others down when they are in need. Sacrifice for others. Keep going.
2. Resonance: As she resonates with this emotional handle, she has the following reactions (body, thoughts, feelings, and impulses to action). Emily feels heaviness in her heart as she attunes to the client. She feels a kind of stuckness when she attunes to the client's dilemma. She resonates with a kind of tightness that feels almost panicky, realizing she has no solution at all for the client caught between so many people she wants to help and feels she must help. No possibility of noticing her own exhaustion ahead of her mother or her staff. She feels an action tendency to want to help Joy slow down to notice her own exhaustion.
3. Emily feels drawn to the client – with a mix of compassion for the weight of responsibility that she carries and admiration for her commitment to her values.
4. Curiosity: Curbing her readiness to assume that the client needs to do things differently and needs to find ways to be assertive and not so bound to want to please others, Emily is eager to be humbly curious to learn more about Joy's Christian faith and her African American culture. She feels limited in fully understanding her "keep going, never mind my own exhaustion and burnout" as connected to her African American identity and to her faith.

Your Strengths and Discoveries about Empathic Attuning

_____

_____

EFIT Empathic Attunement Workout 3: Max, Lingering Guilt and Fear

Context

Max struggles with guilt related to the death of his good friend who was killed in a street-racing crash. A key struggle for him is his disingenuousness and how he has tried to pretend he was not driving the car that crashed, despite the time he spent in jail for criminal negligence causing death. While he developed a career as a meteorologist, appearing successful to the outside world, many struggles with depression and anxiety have filled his private world. He feels he has lived a duplicitous life for the past nearly 30 years and continues to feel paralyzed by fears of remembering the accident scene.

Client Expression

MAX: (Monotone voice with little expression talks about the street-racing crash where he was driving and his passenger was killed.) I never, ever really addressed what happened – it was too painful to face. I developed a series of things that I used to explain away my blame, my fault, my guilt. (Looks up briefly and quickly averts his eyes.) I'd say we were in a head-on collision that took his life and badly injured me and our friend. I would never acknowledge to myself that I was driving nor to anyone that we were street-racing. I'd say we were leaving a party because it looked like there was going to be violence if we didn't get out of there. So, I used things like that to make it look like I was doing the right thing – but really the right thing would have been not to race, in the first place. (Drops his head and gazes at the floor.)

Your Inner Process and Attunement

1. Emotional handle: _____
2. Your internal resonance (body, thoughts, feelings): _____
   _____
3. Do your reactions pull you close or pull you away from Max? _____
4. Area of empathic curiosity to help you to enter more fully into the client's world: _____
   _____

Emily's Inner Process and Attunement

1. Emily identifies as an emotional handle: Max drops his eyes – as he tells her about this moment that has been "too painful to face" and how he looks briefly at her and quickly away again as he says the words, "to explain away my blame, my fault."
2. As she resonates with this emotional handle, she has the following reactions (body, thoughts, feelings, and impulses to action).
   Body: Emily feels tension in her own chest and a weight in her stomach.

Meanings: Emily hears integrity in his clear expression that he tried to excuse his guilt and acknowledges that what he did was wrong.

Feelings: Emily feels compassion for the client carrying blame, fault, shame, and responsibility for this trauma that is decades old and yet alive today.

Impulses to action: Emily wants to validate him for his present-moment integrity – and to help him to tell her his story and to openly face what happened.

3. Her reactions pull her: Emily finds herself drawing close to make it safe to face the pain he has been avoiding; also feels herself drawing back just a little – from what he is finding so very difficult to face. Her fear – will he become overwhelmed? Can I support him and keep him within his window of tolerance?

4. Curiosity: Curbing her readiness to assume she can *fully* understand, she identifies what she is curious to discover: Emily hears that Max feels responsible for his friend's death; his looking away and down while mentioning this, suggests to her that he continues to feel shame and guilt. She feels empathic curiosity about his present-moment experience and about how to make it safe for him to tell his story and to face what has been too difficult to face thus far.

Your Strengths and Discoveries about Empathic Attuning

_____

_____

EMPATHIC REFLECTIONS

Communicating accurate empathic understanding of a client's present-moment process helps a client to feel deeply understood and has the impact of evoking more engagement with their experience. The essence of EFT is, to the best of one's ability, to use one's *empathic imagination* to hear, honor, and get a *felt sense* of another's experience and then to find words to communicate back to the client this *felt sense* understanding. Acknowledging the limits to one's empathic imagination, internally or with the client, is to respect context and culture. When we cannot imagine another's world, we curiously invite more descriptions from the client. It is important to acknowledge, internally or with the client, our limitations at empathically stepping into their world. Slowing down, being tentative, and empathically curious privileges clients' stories and conveys therapist humility. It guards against therapists presuming to understand clients' lived experience and conveying to clients, from an expert or power position, "I know how you feel."

Empathic reflections that communicate accurate understanding are both regulating and evocative, deepening clients' engagement with their own experience. Therapists, however, need to honor the contextual limits of their empathic imaginations and be slow, sensitive, tentative, and curious about clients' responses, and adept at inviting more from the client.

Tentativeness in empathic reflections and explicit invitations for clients to confirm or disconfirm the therapist's communicated understanding engenders a collaborative process for a client to safely bring their story to life in new ways in this interpersonal context. In order to privilege clients as experts of their own stories, *evocative invitations and questions,* explored in later *workouts,* are important micro-skills to fluidly integrate with empathic reflections.

Goals of Empathic Reflection

To communicate an accurate understanding of and resonance with the client.

To convey an invitation for the client to correct, adjust, or confirm the accuracy of that understanding.

To help the client get a *felt sense* of the message they have sent and feel safe to further explore their experience.

To Form an Empathic Reflection

- **Attune** – Imaginatively step into the world of another. <u>Hint</u>: Look for a prominent *emotional or cultural handle*. (See Box 12.2 in *Stepping into Emotionally Focused Therapy*.) Emotional and cultural handles can be offered non-verbally, such as a gulp, facial muscles dropping, eyes narrowing, or any fleeting emotional response briefly evident in facial, bodily, or vocal shifts. They can also be put forward verbally in a poignant phrase or image, such as *injustice; performing blackness; like a broken pitcher; a white marble wall with nothing to hold on to; tugging at my pant leg; caught in the crossfire; a knock on the door.*
- **Resonate** in your own body with the most poignant, most important, most emotionally charged part of the client's non-verbal and verbal message. Pause to notice your cultural or contextual limitations to attune.
- **Find the words**, being mindful of the contextual limits of your empathic imagination. Stay close to or use the client's words to best convey your felt understanding of what the client has conveyed, matching prosody/emotional intensity, <u>*including any themes of attachment or cultural threat/danger.*</u> (Resist inferences and conjectures.)
- **Check with client.** Confirm that your choice of words fits for the client or whether they have a different way of capturing their precise experience, after hearing your words. You can check verbally ("Yes?" Or "Am I getting it?") or with non-verbal tentativeness (through voice inflection), thereby inviting the client to adjust, correct, or confirm your communicated empathic understanding.

Attune to Themes of Threat

Basic attachment threats are nuances of attachment threats of abandonment (a hyperactivating pursuer's worst fear) or of rejection, annihilation, or suffocation (a deactivating, defended withdrawer's worst fear).

Examples of meanings that convey attachment threat include:

- You don't want me.
- You are leaving me.
- You are turning away from me.
- You are judging me as unacceptable.
- You are trying to change me.
- You are despising me.
- You don't care about me.
- I am not important to you.
- I don't matter to you.

Examples of cultural threats include:

- If I express anger or assertiveness I'm judged as "angry" and not to be listened to.
- If I speak up, I might be shot.
- If I simply appear I might be shot or arrested for appearing.
- Cultural attitudes that evaluate personal worth based on skin tone.

The biggest cultural threats are the subtle, unconscious acts of discrimination and marginalization from dominant groups.

How to Form Empathic Reflections

1. **Attune:** Imaginatively step into the world of another. Do you have limitations to your attunement? If so, what are they? Identify the most poignant *emotional/cultural* handle and/or hints of threat to which you attune. Consider whether you need to go back to the previous attunement *workout* for more practice in attuning. Those muscles need practice!
2. **Resonate:** How do you resonate in your own body with the most poignant part of the story?
3. **Find the words** or use the client's words to express your understanding, with tentativeness.
4. **Check with Client:** Invite the client verbally ("Yes?" or, "Am I getting it?") or with non-verbal tentativeness through voice inflection to adjust, correct, or confirm your communicated empathic understanding.

EFCT Empathic Reflection Workouts

EFCT Empathic Reflection Workout 1: José and Phoebe in Early Session

Context
This is an early session with José and Phoebe. Their goals are still unclear and their positions of pursuing and withdrawing remain ambiguous.

Client Expression

JOSÉ: We have times where things are good and then we have very dark times where things are very bad. It's very tough, because we don't hate each other, but we've grown apart in some way.

Your Inner Process and Attunement

1. Attune: Imaginatively step into the world of another. Do you have limitations to your attunement? If so, what are they? _____

_____

2. *Emotional/cultural* handle: Identify the most poignant *emotional/cultural* handle and/or hints of threat to which you attune: _____

_____

3. Bodily resonance: How do you resonate in your own body with the most poignant part of the story?

_____

_____

Your Empathic Reflection
Create an empathic reflection, using words from the emotional handle you have chosen and your own bodily-felt resonance. Communicate your understanding of the client's experience with tentativeness, to invite the client, verbally or with tone of voice to confirm or adjust:

_____

_____

_____

After inserting your empathic reflection, read it out loud.

Emily's Inner Process and Attunement

1. <u>Attune/Limitations</u>: Emily imaginatively steps into the world of José and Phoebe, sensing her limitations to attune to what "not hating each other" feels like for José or how it feels for Phoebe to hear this expression.
2. <u>Emotional handle</u>: Emily chooses these words as the most poignant emotional handle, signaling attachment threat: Some very dark times – grown apart.
3. <u>Bodily resonance</u>: Emily feels a churning, sense of a difficult, lonely struggle.

Emily's Empathic Reflection
(With tentativeness, to invite the client to confirm or adjust her communicated understanding.) Very difficult to have some good times and then some very dark times. It bothers you very much that you have grown so far apart, when you can still feel there is some goodwill between you, yes?

Note: ("Goodwill" is a concrete reframe for *don't hate.*) Emotional handles and phrases in the negative, such as "don't hate" are not something we can empathize with. The absence of an emotion is not concrete, vivid, or specific – the area in which EFT always seeks to work. We cannot empathize with or get a clear feel for what *not hating* feels like. *Don't hate* cannot be framed as something that is tangible. The absence of something cannot be imagined, seen, or felt: Just as we cannot not think of a white elephant nor can we conceptualize *not hating, not being depressed*, or not being *crazy*.

Your Strengths and Discoveries
Compare your inner process and empathic reflection with Emily's. Your responses may be similar or very different from hers and that is ok. Make a note of your strengths at empathic reflecting that you want to celebrate and/or a note of what you may want to add to your practice. The important thing is to experiment with attuning and resonating to get a felt sense of the client's experience and from that resonance to find words to communicate accurate empathic understanding with tentativeness and by inviting the client's response. How did you communicate with tentativeness to invite the client to confirm or adjust your communicated understanding? Your efforts at attuning

and communicating your understanding with tentativeness help clients get a *felt sense* of the message they have sent and feel safe to further explore their experience.

_____

_____

_____

EFCT Empathic Reflection Workout 2: Philip and Precious, How Tradition Matters

Context

Philip and Precious, first-generation immigrants from Zimbabwe have lived in Canada for ten years. Both are successful professionals. Precious, a successful accountant, initiated therapy, because she is concerned about Philip's growing disinterest in her and in the family. In an early session the therapist, with some familiarity with Zimbabwe culture had said to them, "I know this can be a difficult topic to discuss for lots of couples – but I wonder if you can each say something about where you fall in terms of wanting traditional gender roles."

Client Expression

PHILIP: It is hard to say tradition matters – I hate to say it – but it does. (Pauses.) If I am truly honest, I want her to be a traditional wife! (Looks at his professionally dressed wife and hangs his head.) Well, I know that isn't fair to say. (He twists his face and his foot begins to agitate.) She is a successful accountant after all. I wish you hadn't asked. I'd like to take that back.

Your Inner Process and Attunement

1. Attunement and limitations: _____

_____

2. *Emotional/cultural* handle: _____
3. Bodily resonance: _____

Your Empathic Reflection

_____

_____

Emily's Inner Process and Attunement

1. <u>Attune</u>: Emily imaginatively steps into Philip and Precious' world, sensing the following limitation: She senses she has invited Philip to disclose what he now wishes he had not shared. She feels limited in understanding what this has triggered and how it is impacting both Philip and Precious. She feels limited in understanding Philip's regret at admitting that tradition matters to him, and she also recognizes a limitation in understanding what and how tradition is important to him. She is also curious if this is an ongoing argument for them or if they have shared this topic before with no resolution and she is curious if Philip holds back other things that matter a lot to him.

2. Emotional handle: Emily chooses these words as the most poignant *emotional handle*: "I want her to be a traditional wife," followed by, "I wish I hadn't said that."

3. Bodily resonance: Emily feels her body cringing as she realizes she has touched a hot button. She hears Philip regretting what he said, and she gets butterflies in her stomach as she wonders if this is going to evoke an outburst from Precious.

Emily's Empathic Reflection

EMILY: There is something so difficult about acknowledging that tradition is important for you. It's like you admitted something and then immediately are uncomfortable and wish you'd never said it, is that it?

Your Strengths and Discoveries about Empathic Reflection

_____

_____

_____

EFCT Empathic Reflection Workout 3: Peter and Jane, A Stew of Anger

Context

Peter and Jane have recently relocated to a new city, having left behind a bankrupt business. They are getting themselves re-established financially as they have both found employment in their areas of expertise. *Peter* a regular participant in two 12-step groups has been sober for eight months. He continues to struggle with self-doubts and tends to withdraw before speaking up to Jane. When he withdraws and becomes quiet, Jane fears he is upset with he

Client Expression

PETER: I don't know how to communicate with her (shaking head, looking troubled). I just re-play all these things in my head and cook up a stew of anger.

Your Inner Process and Attunement

1. Attunement and limitations: _____

_____

2. *Emotional/cultural* handle: _____

3. Bodily resonance: _____

Your Empathic Reflection

Create an empathic reflection, using words from the emotional handle and your own bodily-felt resonance. Communicate your understanding with tentativeness. Invite the client, verbally or with tone of voice, to confirm or adjust: _____

_____

Emily's Inner Process and Attunement

1. <u>Attune</u>: Emily imaginatively steps into Peter and Jane's world, sensing the following limitation: She senses Peter's concern with holding things in and getting more and more angry in his silence. She recognizes she is limited in understanding how much of a pull Peter feels between the bonds with this 12-step group members and his shaky sense of self and bond with Julie.
2. <u>Emotional handle</u>: Emily chooses these words as the most poignant *emotional handle*: "replaying things in my head" and "cooking up a stew of anger" in combination with the troubled look on his face and his shaking head.
3. <u>Bodily resonance</u>: Emily feels in her body a dizzying sense of being trapped with messages that bother him and growing pressure with an increasing sense of something is not right – no words – just anger.

Emily's Empathic Reflection

You shake your head as you say all these things replay in your head and keep growing into a stew that you don't know how to share with Jane. All that growing pressure and not knowing how to share with Jane, builds and builds into a stew of anger, yes? Something feels not right – no words – just anger, am I understanding?

Your Strengths and Discoveries about Empathic Reflecting

_____

_____

_____

EFCT Empathic Reflection Workout 4: Michael and Jamal, Rebuilding a Tattered Connection

Context

Michael and Jamal are a cisgender, gay couple. Michael recognizes his tendency to turn away from his partner Jamal when he is feeling stressed. He has recently joined a SMART online recovery group (Self-Management and Recovery Training) and they are eager to rebuild their tattered connection.

Client Expression

MICHAEL: I don't talk with Jamal about my gambling, that's true. But I don't want it to be a crutch for "that's the problem with our relationship." I'm not saying it's not part of the pie. It is a big piece of the pie, I'll admit that, but I don't think it's the whole pie. I know I need to find a way to talk more with him… I really do not know how to talk with him anymore, but I want to!

Your Inner Process and Attunement

1. Attunement/Limitations: _____

_____

2. *Emotional/cultural* handle: _____

_____

3. Your bodily resonance: _____

Your Empathic Reflection

_____

_____

After inserting your reflection, read it aloud.

Emily's Inner Process and Attunement

1. Attunement/Limitations: Emily imaginatively steps into Michael's world, sensing the following limitation: She is not clear how much Michael is consumed by his gambling.
2. Emotional handle: Emily chooses these words as the most poignant *emotional handle*: "Not a crutch;" "big piece of the pie;" and "need to talk more with him."
3. Resonance: Emily feels a tug in her own heart as she listens to Michael's sincerity in owning that his gambling does interfere with his relationship with Jamal, and that he doesn't want to use his addictive behavior as an excuse but wants to find a way to share with Jamal.

Emily's Empathic Reflection

EMILY: You know your gambling has a big effect on your relationship and you also know you don't want to use it as an excuse. You clearly want to find a way to be more open with Jamal, do I hear you correctly?

Your Strengths and Discoveries about Empathic Reflecting

_____

_____

_____

EFIT Empathic Reflection Workouts

If you are starting with the EFIT section of the empathic reflection workouts, it is recommended that you first read the introduction to empathic reflection preceding the EFCT empathic reflection workouts, a few pages back.

EFIT Empathic Reflection Workout 1: Levi, Quarantining Emotions

Context

This is an early session with Levi, a Caucasian, cisgender male, in a long-term relationship, struggling with depression and unemployment. His goals are still unclear, though his strategy of de-activating to regulate his emotions has been identified, as is apparent in his expressive images below.

Client Expression

LEVI: I feel like I've been trying to hold everything together for so long – to keep myself from falling apart – pulling all these emotions into a safe corner of myself – to quarantine them. If they weren't quarantined, they would be too much to handle and then the rest of my life would fall apart. I've got to hold everything together; like trying to contain a jack-in-the-box. (He presses his hands down towards the floor.)

Your Inner Process and Attunement

1. Attunement/Limitations: Imaginatively step into the world of another. Do you have limitations to your attunement? If so, what are they? _____
_____

2. *Emotional/cultural* handle: Identify the most poignant *emotional/cultural* handle and/or hints of attachment/cultural threat or safety: _____

3. Bodily resonance: How do you resonate in your own body with the most poignant part of the story? _____

Your Empathic Reflection
Create an empathic reflection, combining words from the emotional handle you have chosen and your own bodily-felt resonance. Communicate your understanding of the client's experience with tentativeness, to invite the client to confirm or adjust: _____
_____
_____

Emily's Inner Process and Attunement

1. Attunement/Limitations: Emily imaginatively steps into Levi's world, recognizing her limitation to fully attune to how emotions can be terrifying for a person. She is also curious to understand more about the pressure of trying to hold back so much that he knows is there.
2. Emotional/cultural handle: Emily chooses these words as the most poignant *emotional handle*: hold everything in a safe corner – if his emotions weren't quarantined, they would be too much to handle; dangerous, like a jack-in-the-box about to pop out. She hears that his own emotions feel threatening.
3. Bodily resonance: Emily resonates in her body with a sense of pressure in her head and a sense of an ominous threat in her chest.

Emily's Empathic Reflection

EMILY: (With a tentative tone, to invite Levi to confirm or adjust her communicated understanding.) Holding it all together – it seems so dangerous to feel all these emotions you are quarantining in that safe corner. So much pressure like a jack-in-a-box. Don't even dare to notice my emotions. Keep the lid on! Am I getting it?

Your Strengths and Discoveries about Empathic Reflecting
Compare your inner process and empathic reflection with Emily's. Your responses may be similar or very different from hers and that is ok.

How did you communicate with tentativeness to invite the client to confirm or adjust your communicated understanding?

Your efforts at attuning and communicating your understanding with tentativeness help clients get a *felt sense* of the message they have sent and feel safe to further explore their experience. Make a note of your strengths at empathic reflecting that you want to celebrate and/or a note of what you may want to add to your practice. The important thing is to experiment with attuning and resonating to get a felt sense of the client's experience, and from that resonance, to find words to communicate accurate empathic understanding with tentativeness and by inviting the client's response.

_____

_____

_____

EFIT Empathic Reflection Workout 2: Neil, Unexpected Loss and Anger

Context

Neil is a single white cisgender man in his late fifties struggling with an unexpected relationship breakup. As he tells the story of having expected the relationship he was in to be long-term, he fluctuates between brief tears, physical trembling, and talk of anger.

Client Expression

NEIL: (Trembling and in tears.) Dora and I spoke for years of growing old together, and I expected we still had a long life ahead of us, so it came totally out of the blue when she told me she is leaving! I am crushed. I feel it physically (He motions from his stomach up to his throat – wringing his hands – looking in desperation at the therapist. Suddenly, he flicks off his tears. He curls his fingers into a fist and then throws up his hands in a gesture of helplessness.) It scares me to see what will happen if I let my anger out – like why didn't she give me more warning? Why did she decide to leave? She says there is no one else – just didn't feel our relationship was working. It makes no sense! This is a lot of anger for one person to handle – alone!

Your Inner Process and Attunement

1. Attunement/Limitations: _____

_____

2. *Emotional/cultural* handle: _____
3. Bodily resonance: _____

Your Empathic Reflection

_____

_____

Emily's Inner Process and Attunement

1. Attunement/Limitations: Emily feels her heart clench as she resonates to his tears, which he brushes off as quickly as they come; she clenches her own fist, mirroring his frustration at this unexpected news, resonating with his very legitimate anger and apparent helplessness at this

shattering announcement from his wife, Dora. She feels some twinges of helplessness at how to support him in his overwhelming grief, particularly when his tears are rapidly replaced with anger at this sudden loss that is shaking his whole world. She realizes she may have some limitations in attuning to someone significantly older than her. Another limitation she senses is that she, herself, has not lived with a fear of her anger being too much to manage, yet she hears that is a core theme for Neil.

2. *Emotional/cultural handle*: What strikes Emily as the most poignant emotional handles are his words, "Why did she have to leave? My anger scares me. It is a lot of anger for one person to handle." And his bodily signals; brushing off his tears, his tightened fist, and his hands thrown up in what looks to her sign a sign of defeat or helplessness.

3. Bodily resonance: Her heart swells with compassion and respect and a need to be fully present as she resonates with his enormous loss and with his attachment fear of managing his own anger alone. One person alone with outrage is scary! She feels much respect for this man who can actually say that it is too much anger to handle. She feels herself pulling close to make it safe for his anger, and his tears that he has brushed away, to have a voice.

Emily's Empathic Reflection

EMILY: (Mirroring Neil's gesture of a tightened fist.) You know you feel anger at this sudden and expected loss of Dora, the woman you love and never expected would leave you. You are crushed by her announcement! You can make no sense of it and your anger rises and you brush away the tears and the sadness. It is very frightening to feel this anger and not know how to safely express it, yes? It definitely feels too big to handle alone. (Adding the attachment significance.) Am I getting it?

Your Strengths and Discoveries about Empathic Reflection

_____

_____

_____

EFIT Empathic Reflection Workout 3: Hedy, Overthinking Everything

Context

Hedy, an immigrant to the United States, is university-educated and in a professional career. She immigrated five years earlier to marry her husband who had immigrated ahead of her.

Client Expression

HEDY: I over-think everything…. I have a problem with decision-making, I always have second thoughts um…so yeah … Never quite know how I feel. I'm married five years. (Pause, looks down, big sigh.) It's not going well – we might divorce – but I'm going to change my job. (Pace quickens.) Right now, I have a part-time job but… I'm starting a totally new field. I'm starting to study accounting. (Face brightens.) And I like it but I'm still unsure about everything and those thoughts, "Am I doing the right thing?" The troublesome thoughts are coming and going and it's just so bothersome.

Your Inner Process and Attunement

1. Attunement/Limitations: _____

_____

2. *Emotional/cultural* handle: _____

3. Bodily resonance: _____

Your Empathic Reflection

_____

_____

Emily's Inner Process and Attunement

1. Attunement/Limitations: Emily attunes to the uncertainty and chaos that Hedy is describing. She attunes to the facial changes when Hedy speaks of her marriage and her new field of study. She notices a strength – a spark of certainty that she trusts that she chose the right field of study. She is also aware that she is limited in fully understanding Hedy's experience of being in a new land away from her home country.
2. *Emotional/cultural* handle: The most poignant emotional handle she perceives is the sudden change in Hedy's face from speaking of uncertainty and her marriage and the burst of brightness when speaking of her accounting studies.
3. Bodily resonance: Emily feels an openness in her heart to learn more about Hedy's confusion, grief, and decision-making, marked by a sudden joy to see the brightness on Hedy's face as she talks of something she is certain she is happy about.

Emily's Empathic Reflection

EMILY: It sounds like it is so hard to trust yourself, so alone in this new country. Thoughts keep bombarding you and you feel unsure of yourself in many ways. Your face drops and you heave a big sigh as you speak about your marriage and then you brighten up as you say, "I found a field of study that I totally like." That is one thing you are sure about, yes?

Your Strengths and Discoveries about Empathic Reflecting

_____

_____

_____

EFIT Empathic Reflecting Workout 4: Hedy, Immigration Struggles

Context

This workout continues with the same client from the previous workout. Hedy, in her first session, is grieving the end of her short marriage, and describing the loneliness of being an immigrant and her strained connections with her family back in Germany.

Client Expression

HEDY: It is hard to come to this new country all by myself – being alone having no one and having a lot of hope in my husband and how hard it is to have just one person and he disappoints you but, but some days I am more bothered by my family. My family doesn't understand. They just want me to focus on my career. It just hurts. I came here to have love, to have a good relationship and all they can talk about is me getting a better job. They just don't know how much it hurts.

Your Inner Process and Attunement

1. Attunement/Limitations: _____

2. *Emotional/cultural* handle: _____

3. Bodily resonance: _____

Your Empathic Reflection

_____

_____

Emily's Inner Process and Attunement

1. Attunement/Limitations: Emily attunes to Hedy's loneliness and grief in a new country, also the courage it took to immigrate; she tunes into the disappointment of her failed marriage; she also attunes that even more, right now, she is bothered by her family's lack of understanding of her pain. Emily recognizes her limitation to fully feel the grief and loneliness of immigration and living in a new country.
2. *Emotional/cultural* handle: The most poignant *emotional/cultural* handles that strike Emily are *new country – came for love – didn't work – family doesn't understand.*
3. Bodily resonance: Emily resonates with a sense of heaviness and hollowness all at the same time for Hedy's losses, disappointment, loneliness, and emotional pain.

Emily's Empathic Reflection

EMILY: What a huge amount of loss and feeling alone – losing the relationship with your husband that you counted on in this new country! Feeling so misunderstood by your family who seems to totally miss your grief and loneliness, yes?

Your Strengths and Discoveries about Empathic Reflecting

_____

_____

_____

EVOCATIVE RESPONSES AND QUESTIONS FOR ELABORATION

Evocative micro-skills responses and questions are all used to elicit more specificity and granularity of emotional experience, thereby deepening clients' present-moment experience and strengthening the alliance between client and therapist. Evocative micro-skills have various functions and are embedded in Move 1 tracking reflections, are featured in Move 2 assembly and deepening, and are the primary intervention in Move 4 processing, where the therapist asks how it was to share a particular message and how it was to receive that message. In the introduction to Empathic Reflection Workouts, there is an emphasis on integrating evocative questions and responses fluidly with empathic reflections, to privilege clients as experts of their own stories. Hence, in the evocative workouts, you are asked to *make a reflection before evoking*. Skilled EFT therapists will tend, after evoking something new, to reflect the newness again, and then to validate it.

Questions, even evocative questions, can be overused. Reflections, joining with, and validating are more important micro-skills in experiential therapy than asking questions. Also, remember that the primary purpose of evocative questions is to expand and organize the client's emotional experience and enhance empathic understanding.

Evocative interventions can contribute to cultural humility by inviting clients to share their world and story before presuming one can understand a client's nuanced experience in their context. Additionally, evocative responses and questions are used to find focus, formulate specific hopes and goals for therapy, elaborate on emotional experience, patterns, and strategies, and in EFCT, to segue effectively to the partner, throughout therapy and particularly in Move 4 processing to elicit the partner's response. Evocative questions and responses, not included in this workout section, are the many targeted evocative micro-interventions used in the assessment. (See Chapter 7 in *Stepping into Emotionally Focused Therapy* and "A Closer Look at Areas for Assessment and Sample Questions" in the online support material for that chapter, for many of those evocative questions.) Evocative micro-skills used in combination with therapist transparency to build and maintain task alliance are included in the therapist transparency workouts later in Part 1.

How to Evoke to Expand Emotional Experience

As with all micro-skills in this book, a therapist has an inner process of attunement before finding the words to respond.

Therapist Inner Process and Attunement

- **Identify salience:** Ask yourself, "What is the salient part of the message (emotional/cultural handle) to take hold of to elicit elaboration of (attachment/relational) emotional experience?"
- **Identify the explicit elements of emotion** that the client is expressing. For example, what is the cue/trigger that signals a threat? What are the visible somatic reactions (facial or bodily

movements)? What is the client saying about the meanings they are making? What are the client's action tendencies? Are there hints of the core, underlying emotion?

- **Identify missing or vague elements**. For example, you may not know what triggered this emotional cascade, but you know what the client does or feels like doing, or the meaning the client is making. Whatever element the client is familiar with can be your launching pad to join with the client and from there to evoke more elements not yet specified.

Forming an Evocative Response or Question (to Assemble and Specify)

- **Repeat or reflect** a key element that the client has expressed or hinted at, a cultural or emotional handle, to elicit more breadth, depth, and aliveness about this element and/or to evoke missing or hidden elements of emotion.
- **After repeating that emotional handle, choose one of the following:**

  1. A simple reflection: Be silent to allow the client to expand after your simple reflection.
  2. An invitation to expand: Invite the client to expand on what you just repeated.
  3. A question targeted at a specific element of emotion, or a vague or unexpressed element of emotion.

Details on the Three Forms of Evocative Micro-Skills

As noted above, an evocative micro-skill most effectively expands a client's emotional experience and depth when it is preceded with a reflection of something the client has already conveyed. Three options for evoking are detailed below.

1. *Simple reflection (repetition of key client words)*

    An evocative response may be a simple repetition of an emotional handle, poignant phrase, or bodily movement. Repeating the client's words in a slow, soft, simple manner is evocative and, by implication, invites the client to expand. Example: "*No room for me in his world.*" (Words in italics are the client's own words. They are repeated slowly and softly.)

2. *An open invitation to expand in something specific*

    An evocative response may also be a request to say more about something specific that a client has expressed.

    Examples *(Words in italics are the client's own words or somatic signal.)*
    Verbal communication: "Say more about *that difficult time?*"
    Non-verbal: "Can you describe what was happening as *a grimace just crossed your face?*"

3. *Evocative questions targeted at specific elements of emotion*

    Evocative questions can be targeted at a specific element of the emotional process. Words in italics are specific to eliciting different elements of emotion, as noted below:

- To evoke the cue/trigger: *When* do you feel or react like that?
- To evoke the action tendency: *How* do you typically *react?* and *What* do you *do/feel like doing?*
- To evoke the bodily response: *What* does your *body do?* and *Where in your body* do you feel that?
- To evoke the meaning-making: *What does it say* to you? and *What do you say* to yourself?

What to Evoke?

EFT therapists evoke elements of emotion; increase specificity and granularity; and focus on formulating longings and goals. Additionally, evocative micro-skills are used to evoke one partner's response to another partner's disclosure, to elicit examples of a positive cycle or pattern and a description of the typical reactive/coping pattern; to elicit reflections on the experience of encounters (as discloser or as receiver); and finally, to invite clients' overall perspective on a session or therapy process.

1. **Evoke Elements of Emotion**

    Notice which elements of emotion (underlined below) that a client is conveying and which are hidden:

    Is there a limbic perception of threat or safety?

    What is the external/interpersonal cue/trigger?

    Do I see somatic reactions such as facial or bodily movements? Or, Does the client report bodily sensations?

    What meaning is the client making or stating as fact?

    What are the client's action tendencies or emotional reactions (such as getting angry, brushing it off with annoyance and logic, etc.?

    Do I detect hints of core emotion?

    Name elements you hear or see (cue, action, body, meaning, and core fear) in a vivid, specific, concrete manner, linking elements together and matching the client's emotional tone. Replaying the cue is an effective way to evoke more. Repeating the *cultural/emotional handle,* with empathic curiosity evokes expansion. A word is likely to have a nuanced meaning for each client. EFT therapists try to avoid assuming that they understand what someone means by a word they use. *Fear* or *sadness* or *"stay strong,"* for example, all have different, unique meanings for everyone! Some words are the handle opening into an entire story of great import! Questions targeted to specific elements of emotion (see bottom of p. 24), and open-ended questions evoke specificity and granular experience. After evoking a response, EFT therapists take time to reflect on their understanding of the client's response and to check for verbal/non-verbal confirmation that their communicated understanding of the client's responses matches their experience.

2. **Evoke More Specificity and Granularity**

    Vague or impersonal emotional or cultural phrases or non-verbal messages are markers for an EFT therapist to evoke more specificity, granularity, and deeper engagement. This may include moving from past tense to present tense, from recounting past stories to evoking present-moment experience of reliving that story, or moving from speaking generally to the more personal, present. It may also include vague content that needs to be named explicitly, such as hints of an attachment injury, references to socio-cultural contexts and impacts of marginalization, causal comments about sex, addictive processes, violence, or aggression. Recognize when you need help to attune to a cultural experience or context that may be markedly different from your own or when something seems randomly mentioned and then dismissed. These are important doorways not to be missed.

    Showing curiosity and evoking to expand on the content of attachment injuries, cultural or contextual nuances, or any hints of content that appear difficult for clients to discuss, conveys respect. It is not the EFT therapist's job to understand everything about each client. It is our responsibility to be attuned to detect doorways on which we can knock to invite expansion. With the expansion, clients can assemble their emotional experiences more coherently and therapists can understand them more accurately. It is a collaborative process that benefits both the client and the therapist.

Emotional or cultural handles are poignant emotion-filled words, images, metaphors, or bodily movements that a therapist can repeat, to evoke or capture a client's as-yet-unformulated emotions or cultural stories. Like handles on a door, they can be held gently and turned, opening doorways into new, expansive experiences. They are likely to contain many or all the elements of emotion: trigger, body, meaning, action impulse, and core fear. Examples include: *keep on going – you can handle it; traditional role; performing blackness; not a beautiful corpse; stay away from hatred; exclusion; ugly; and superwoman.* EFT therapists repeat the phrase or *emotional/cultural handle* and offer evocative invitations for a client to open the doorway as much as they are willing. To avoid exploring cultural handles is to miss critically important emotions and views of self and other. For example, if a therapist skims past a Black client's casual reference to "our plight" without pausing to invite more, they are ignoring volumes of lived experience that a client may want or be willing to explore.

3. **Evoke to Find Focus, Coherence, and Goals**

   When there is confusion, ambivalence, or distracting content, evoke attachment significance, to focus on what is most important for the client and their survival, and link to previous sessions, longings, and core difficult, dangerous, unacceptable, and foreign emotions, to find clarity and focus on the goals clients have identified.

4. **Additional Elements to Evoke**

   Additionally, evocative micro-skills are used to evoke one partner's response to the other partner's disclosure, to elicit examples of a positive cycle or pattern and a description of the typical reactive/coping pattern; to elicit reflections on the experience of encounters (as discloser or as receiver); and finally, to invite clients' overall perspective on a session or therapy process.

Evocative Micro-Skill Prompts

Therapist Inner Process/Attunement:

1. Ask yourself, "What is the salient part of the message to take hold of to elicit elaboration of (attachment / relational) emotional experience?"
2. Identify the elements of emotion the client is conveying: The cue/trigger that signals a threat? Somatic reactions (facial or bodily movements)? What is the client saying about the meanings they are making? What are the client's action tendencies? Are there hints of the core, underlying emotion?
3. Identify elements that seem to be missing or vague. (For example, you do not know what triggered this emotional cascade; you do not know what the client does or feels like doing.)

Form Evocative Micro-Interventions:

1. Begin with a simple reflection: Repeat a key element that the client has expressed or hinted at, a cultural or emotional handle, to elicit more breadth, depth, and aliveness about this element and/or to evoke missing or hidden elements of emotion.
2. Choose to do one of the following:

   i. Pause to allow the client to expand after your simple reflection.
   ii. Invite the client to expand on what you just repeated. (Tell me more about…)
   iii. Ask a question targeted at a vague or unexpressed element of emotion (such as the evocative questions targeted at specific elements of emotion).

EFCT Evocative Workouts

The four *EFCT evocative workouts* are focused on evoking elements of emotion. These are important micro-skills needed for Move 2, and for other moves as well.

EFCT Evocative Workout 1: Evoking Elements of Emotion with Sophie and Ella, Seeking to Share Safely

Context

Sophie and Ella are a biracial lesbian couple. Ella, the more withdrawn partner, identifies as Chinese Canadian and Sophie, a more anxious pursuer, identifies as white European.

Client Expression

Read the client's expression below aloud as though you were the client. Then follow the prompts to identify your inner attunement process and to create your own evocative response or question to invite elaboration.

SOPHIE: (Takes a big sigh; tone heightens as she speaks.) I don't know how to safely share things that are bothering me without pushing Ella away!

Your Inner Process and Attunement

1. Identify salience (the most emotionally or culturally poignant or striking part of the client's message) for expansion; attune to how this resonates in your own body: _____
2. Identify explicit elements of emotion the client is conveying: _____
3. Identify vague or missing elements of emotion to evoke or specify:_____

Your Evocative Response to Invite Elaboration

1. Reflect/repeat, the salient element, emotional/cultural handle: _____
2. Choose one of the following evocative micro-skills or experiment with all three:
   a. pause to wait for the client to add more to your reflection;
   b. invite the client to say more about the key element you repeated; or

c. ask a question targeted at a specific element of emotion.

_____

_____

_____

After inserting your evocative response or question, read it aloud. Does it invite the client to say more, to expand their engagement?

   Next, compare your responses with Emily's below to see if you discover anything you may want to integrate into your EFT *way of being*.

Emily's Inner Process and Attunement
Read Emily's responses aloud to get a feel for how evocative they sound.

1. Salience: Emily identifies *how to safely share without pushing Ella away* as the most poignant emotional handle. She feels a slight churning in her stomach as she resonates with Sophie's dilemma.
2. Elements conveyed: Emily identifies that Sophie is conveying the following elements of emotion:
     Trigger: Somewhat unclear – likely images of Ella distancing when she shares.
     Action tendency: Wants to talk to Ella about things bothering her.
     Body: Big sigh; heightened tone.
     Meaning: My sharing pushes Ella away.
3. Missing or vague elements of emotion: Emily is curious to evoke more about (i) the trigger for Sophie's sigh; (ii) Sophie's awareness about her action tendency to push Ella away, and to help her own that her best attempts to share do, in fact, have the impact of Ella backing away; and (iii) also curious to evoke more about a core fear implied in "how to safely share."

Emily's Evocative Responses, for Each of the Three Options

1. Reflection: Such a dilemma, "How to safely share without pushing Ella away!" pauses for Sophie to expand.
2. Invitation to expand on her own action tendency: Can you say more about noticing that your best attempts to share with Ella, actually seem to push her away?
    Invitation to expand on the hint of her core fear: Can you say more about how you feel unsafe to share – so afraid Ella will back away?
3. Targeted evocative questions:

   • To evoke the trigger: *When* do you notice Ella begins to back away? Or *What happened just before* you took that big sigh and said your sharing that seems to push Ella away?
   • To evoke her action tendency: What do you *do* when you want to talk to Ella about things that bother you?

Your Strengths and Discoveries
After reading Emily's responses, compare your responses with hers and see if you discover anything you may want to integrate into the style of using evocative micro-skills to expand. Also, make a note of your evocative strengths. Your evocative micro-skills may be similar to Emily's responses or very different – either is ok. The goal here is to practice joining with your clients where they are, recognizing which elements of emotion they have conveyed, and evoking expansion of their experience.

_____

_____

_____

EFCT Evocative Workout 2: Evoking Elements of Emotion with Wayne and Jessica as Contextual Survival Strategies Come Home

Context

Wayne and Jessica have a pursue/withdraw distress cycle, where at times they also both with-draw, although Jessica is more of a pursuer for connection and Wayne is more on guard to avoid upsetting Jessica. Wayne is Black with an Ethiopian heritage and Jessica, with a much lighter skin tone, identifies as white and Argentinian. Some of the exploration with the couple is how the impacts of Wayne's experiences in an office of mostly white colleagues weigh him down and constrict his interactions with Jessica as well.

Client Expression

WAYNE: We are doing ok, I think. Days I work from home are comforting in a way – not being in an office where I have to perform blackness takes a lot of stress off the top of my head.

Your Inner Process and Attunement

1. Identify salience (the most emotionally or culturally poignant or striking part of the client's message) for expansion; attune to how this resonates in your own body: _____
2. Identify explicit elements of emotion the client is conveying: _____
3. Identify vague or missing elements of emotion to evoke or specify: _____

Your Evocative Response to Invite Elaboration

1. Repeat, the emotional/cultural handle: _____
2. Choose one of the following evocative micro-skills or experiment with all three:

   a. pause to wait for the client to add more to your reflection;
   b. invite the client to say more about the key element you repeated; or
   c. ask a question targeted at a specific element of emotion.

   _____

   _____

   _____

Emily's Inner Process and Attunement

1. Salience: Emily identifies *having to perform blackness* and *comforting working from home* as the most poignant emotional/cultural handles. She feels fluttering in her chest as she resonates with this, recognizing her limitations as a white woman to understand the survival pressure of the expectation to "perform blackness."

2. Elements conveyed: Emily identifies that Wayne is conveying the following elements of emotion, and also realizes she is limited in fully understanding Wayne's experience of these elements:

    <u>Trigger</u>: Working from home versus working where he needs to "perform blackness"

    <u>Action tendency</u>: Not "perform blackness."

    <u>Body</u>: Stress in his head is relieved.

    <u>Meaning implied</u>: *Others expect something from me; my survival depends on performing a certain way.*

3. Missing or vague elements of emotion: Emily is curious to evoke more about what "performing blackness" means to Wayne and also what "not performing blackness from the comfort of home" is like. As a white woman, she cannot presume to understand his experience. She is also curious about how much his wife understands. Finally, she is curious about Wayne's bodily experience of relief and how he experiences that in his relationship with Jessica.

Emily's evocative responses, for each of the three options.

Continue to read your and Emily's responses aloud to get a feel for how evocative they sound.

1. <u>Reflection</u>: Emily reflects slowly, and softly, "Working from home has lifted the stress of having to perform blackness?" with inflection as a question, and then pauses to make room for Wayne to say more about that experience.

2. <u>Invitation to expand</u> (several examples):

    I hear working from home has lifted some of your stress. Help me and Jessica understand what having to *perform blackness* means for you.

    Can you tell me more about the comfort of working from home?

    Help me understand how the relief of "not having to perform blackness at work" may impact you at home with Jessica.

3. <u>Targeted evocative questions</u>, targeted at specific elements of emotion:

    To evoke the <u>action tendency</u>, Emily reflects "Having to perform blackness. What is it that you do differently in the moments to perform blackness?

    To evoke <u>action tendency</u> in a relationship: How are you able to share with Jessica about this relief? Or about the comfort of working from home?

    To evoke his <u>bodily experience</u>: What does this "relief in your head" without having to perform blackness feel like in your body?

Your Strengths and Discoveries about Evocative Responding

_____

_____

_____

EFCT Evocative Workout 3: Evoking Elements of Emotion with Will and Priscilla During Stage 2 Engagement

Context

Will and Priscilla have de-escalated their pursue/withdraw distress cycle in Stage 1 and are moving into Stage 2. Will is becoming more comfortable having a voice in place of his former pattern of avoiding conflict until he blurts out a barrel of resentments. Priscilla appreciates hearing more from Will and is happy they can have some disagreements without Will bolting away in disgust. Will has disclosed his fears to Priscilla that she will get fed up with him again, that he fears he can never do enough to make her happy with him, that she is really trying to make him into someone he can never be, and that she can never accept and appreciate him for who he is. She has responded with surprise and somewhat reluctant acceptance of Will's newly disclosed fears. In processing this fear with the therapist, Will has identified the need embedded in his fear of Priscilla getting fed up and pressuring him to be different: He longs for her acceptance and to know she likes him. In this moment, the therapist is helping Will to shape a reach to Priscilla to ask for what he needs to stay engaged.

Client Expression

WILL: I do want to keep showing up more. It's so much better being seen and heard in this relationship. I want to keep having an impact on what happens between us. (He takes a quick glance at Priscilla who has a frown.) But… (Shrugs his shoulders, looks out the window, and stops talking.)

Your Inner Process and Attunement

1. Identify salient elements to expand; attune to how this resonates in your own body:

_____

2. Identify explicit elements of emotion the client is conveying: _____

_____

3. Identify vague or missing elements of emotion to evoke or specify: _____

Your Evocative Response to Invite Elaboration

1. Reflect/repeat, the salient element, emotional/cultural handle: _____
2. Choose one of the following evocative micro-skills or experiment with all three:

   a. pause to wait for the client to add more to your reflection;
   b. invite the client to say more about the key element you repeated; or
   c. ask a question targeted at a specific element of emotion.

_____

_____

_____

Emily's Inner Process and Attunement

1. Salience: Emily identifies *I want to keep showing up; I want to keep having an impact, but ...* as the most poignant emotional/cultural handles; after seeing Priscilla's frown, Will stops speaking, shrugs, and looks away. Emily feels her heart sink. Her hopefulness in facilitating this important request-encounter is put on pause.
2. Elements conveyed: Emily identifies the following elements of emotion for Will.
   Trigger: Priscilla's frown.
   Action tendencies and obvious bodily reactions: began to risk asserting himself, checked Priscilla's face, shrugged his shoulder, stopped speaking, and looked away.
3. Missing or vague elements of emotion: Emily is curious to evoke more about the meaning he made of the frown on Priscilla's face. She is also eager to evoke or refocus him on the core fear in this rapid cascade of *trigger-feeling-meaning-stopped-talking* process.

Emily's evocative responses to invite elaboration of Will's present-moment experience, to continue to shape the encounter.

1. Reflection: Emily reflects slowly in a proxy voice, "I want to keep showing up. This is so much better, BUT ---?" ... Then pauses for Will to say more about that experience.
2. Invitation to expand (with a replay of the trigger and process): You were about to ask Priscilla for what you need from her to remain as engaged as you have been, when suddenly you checked her face and stopped yourself. Can you tell me what just came up as you looked at Priscilla and shrugged?
3. Targeted evocative questions (Several examples):
   To expand on trigger and meaning: What did you see on Priscilla's face that stopped you in your tracks?
   To evoke and refocus Will on experiencing his core fear and its embedded need:
   Notice what is happening in your body as you just turned away from the person whose acceptance you crave.
   What is happening in your body that says, "Stop, don't dare ask"
   To evoke and validate the riskiness of the action tendency to make a request of Priscilla: So difficult to ask Priscilla to accept you and like you, yes?

Your Strengths and Discoveries about Evocative Responding

_____

_____

_____

EFCT Evocative Workout 4: Evoking Elements of Emotion with Will and Priscilla During a Softening

Context
Will and Priscilla have completed the engagement change event. Will is clearly engaged and Priscilla's anxiety seems as intense as ever. She doesn't know if it is safe to trust he will remain engaged, but

she is beginning to experience he is "truly in." Her view of other is stabilizing. She is trusting he is accessible, responsive, and engaged, however, this is triggering self-doubts and self-loathing. She describes her view of self as pathetic, needy, and "shameful that I was such a monster all these years." The therapist is helping her to shape an encounter to share this clearly distilled fear of being a pathetic monster in Will's eyes. In the midst of disclosing this fear at a high level of experience, Priscilla halts, appears flooded, and needs help to come back to a manageable emotional window of tolerance.

Client Expression

PRISCILLA: Will, it's hard to look at you, feeling like this pathetic, needy monster. All this shrieking – so panicked whenever you would go away… so afraid you see me as too much. (Looks at Will, and he is looking back softly and kindly.) Well, I was too much… I am too much. (Twisting tissue between her fingers; drops her face in her hands, weeping; Will wraps his arm around her shoulder, and she leans into him.)

Your Inner Process and Attunement

1. Identify the most emotionally or culturally poignant part of the client's message for expansion; attune to how this resonates in your own body: _____
2. Identify explicit elements of emotion conveyed: _____
3. Identify vague or missing elements of emotion to evoke: _____

Your Evocative Response to Invite Elaboration

1. Repeat, the salient element, emotional/cultural handle: _____
2. Choose one of the following evocative micro-skills or experiment with all three:

   a. pause to wait for the client to add more to your reflection;
   b. invite the client to say more about the key element you repeated; or
   c. ask a question targeted at a specific element of emotion.

   _____

   _____

   _____

Emily's Inner Process and Attunement

1. Salience: Emily identifies *Will moving close and putting his arm around Priscilla while she weeps in fear that she is too much for him; Priscilla saying, "hard to look at Will,"* as the most poignant emotional/cultural handles. Emily feels a mix of Priscilla's fear and weight of shame with a burning warmth and excitement in her heart at the image of Will confidently moving close to Priscilla in tears. This is new!
2. Elements conveyed: Emily identifies that Priscilla has conveyed the following elements of emotion:

   Trigger: Will's presence.
   Body: Twisting fingers, weeping, and hiding face.

Meanings: I am a pathetic monster, I am too much for Will.
Action tendency: Tells Will she is too much.

3. Missing or vague elements of emotion: Emily is curious to evoke more about Priscilla's present-moment experience as she has just disclosed to Will her deepest fear that she is too much for him, and he has moved close to her. This is noteworthy, confirming his engagement, which is unlike his typical move in their cycle which was to pull away whenever Priscilla flooded with tears.

Emily's Evocative Responses to Invite Elaboration. (First reflects, then evokes)

1. Reflection: Emily reflects slowly, "You just disclosed to Will your deepest fear that you are too much for him, and he moved right in and put his arm around you!" Pauses to allow Priscilla to describe the experience.
2. Invitation to expand: Emily reflects, "You just disclosed to Will your deepest fear that you are too much for him, and he moved right in and put his arm around you! Just notice in your body how it is to have him holding you close in this frightening moment."
   Or, "How is it for you that your tears and words of embarrassment that he would see you as a monster are not pushing him away but pulling him close to protect and soothe you?"
3. Targeted evocative questions:
   To evoke meaning: Emily reflects, "You just disclosed to Will your deepest fear that you are too much for him, and he moved right in and put his arm around you! What does that say to you about how Will sees you?" (to evoke her present-moment meaning-making).
   To evoke expansion of Priscilla's core fear: "All these years of fighting to pull Will close and now he is here responding to you as you tell him you might be too much for him. What is your fear – the fear that stopped you from talking to him just now – what is it saying?"

Your Strengths and Discoveries about Evocative Responding

_____

_____

_____

The online support material has more evocative workouts to invite specificity and granularity and to find focus and elicit goals. (See routledge.com/9781032151311)

EFIT Evocative Workouts

If you are beginning with the EFIT evocative workouts, be sure to read the introduction given before the EFCT evocative workouts. It contains much relevant information that will help to guide you through the EFIT evocative workouts as well.

When exploring ways to evoke more of the client's emotional experience, it is often helpful to tune into an emotional handle or specific element of emotion as a launching pad from which to evoke other elements (trigger, bodily arousal, meaning made, reactive emotion/action tendency, and hints of core, underlying emotion). Typically, emotional handles (images, phrases) contain all elements of emotion once they are assembled. For your practice and attunement, you are asked to identify all the elements of emotion you can for each of the workouts in this section, even if you do not draw on all the elements to expand, create coherence, or find focus.

EFIT Evocative Workout 1: Evoking to Elaborate, with Joy

Context

Joy, whom you met in the empathic attunement workout, is a young professional, identifying as Christian and Black African American. She is experiencing fatigue with work demands and with supporting her family emotionally and financially.

Client Expression

JOY: I don't know if my mother is staying with my father just for the sake of having someone there to call a partner or if she's afraid to walk away from the relationship. Growing up, I witnessed him being abusive to her. She never said much, but now, quite often, I get pulled into the situations that are going on between her and my father and she uses me as a sounding board. She confides in me when things are going badly between them. There is a part of me that feels there's a line that should be there and that she shouldn't cross because even though she can talk to me, that's still my father, so there's certain discussions or certain topics that I should not be brought into, but she tends to treat me more like a friend, as opposed to a daughter. (Smiles and then heaves a big sigh!)

Your Inner Process and Attunement

1. Emotion/cultural handle to expand; resonate in your own body: _____
_____
2. Explicit elements of emotion: _____
3. Vague or missing elements of emotion to evoke: _____

Your Evocative Responses to Invite Elaboration

1. Repeat, the salient element, emotional/cultural handle: _____
2. Choose one of the following evocative micro-skills or experiment with all three:

   a. reflect and pause to wait for the client to add more to your reflection,
   b. invite the client to say more about the key element you repeated, or
   c. ask a question targeted at a specific element of emotion:

   _____

   _____

   _____

Emily's Inner Process and Attunement

1. Salience: Emily identifies *uses me, crosses a line, more like a friend than a daughter* as salient emotional handles. Emily's heart feels heavy with a sense of being leaned on by so many people without receiving nurturing in return.
2. Elements of emotion conveyed: Emily identifies that Joy is conveying:
   A <u>trigger</u> is that mother confides and "uses" her as a sounding board; crosses a line.
   <u>Meanings</u>: There is a line that mother should not cross; she shares too much with me; she uses me as a friend, not a daughter.
   <u>Action tendency</u>: I get pulled into conversations I don't like.
3. Missing or vague elements of emotion: Emily is curious to evoke more about Joy's action impulse (what she feels like doing) in this experience of *being used* and having her mother *cross this line*. She is also curious to elicit Joy's bodily-felt sense and more specifics of her image of longing to be treated like a daughter.

Emily's Evocative Responses to Invite Elaboration. (First reflects, then evokes.)

1. <u>Reflection</u>:
   Emily: (Reflecting slowly) Very stressful when you want your parents to be your parents… Then she pauses to allow Joy to say more.
2. <u>Invitation to expand (on the action impulse)</u>:
   Emily: Very stressful when you want your parents to be your parents! Tell me more about how you cope with your mother leaning on you like this.
3. <u>Targeted questions</u>:
   To evoke the <u>action tendency</u>: When you experience that your mother leans on you more than you want, and treats you like a friend more than a daughter, what do you feel like doing?
   To evoke her <u>bodily-felt sense</u>: Where in your body do you feel this sense of longing to be your mother's daughter, not a friend?

Your Strengths and Discoveries about Evocative Responding

_____

_____

_____

EFIT Evocative Workout 2: Joy, Expanding from an Image

Context (Same client as above):

Client Expression

JOY: I feel like a pitcher. Like a pitcher for water or juice or soda or whatever, and I pour from my pitcher into everybody's cup when they need to be filled up, but when my pitcher is empty, instead of me taking the time to fill up my own pitcher, when people still need, even though

I don't have to give, I start to chip away pieces of my pitcher instead of taking that time to uh, make sure that I am okay and I am taking care of myself and refilling my own pitcher.

Your Inner Process and Attunement

1. Salience for expansion; resonate in your own body: _____
2. Explicit elements of emotion: _____
3. Vague or missing elements of emotion to evoke or specify: _____

Your Evocative Responses to Invite Elaboration

1. Repeat, the salient element, emotional/cultural handle: _____
2. Choose one of the following evocative micro-skills or experiment with all three:

   a. reflect and pause to wait for the client to add more to your reflection,
   b. invite the client to say more about the key element you repeated, or
   c. ask a question targeted at a specific element of emotion:

   _____

   _____

   _____

   _____

Emily's Inner Process and Attunement

1. Salience: Emily identifies the *empty pitcher* and *chipping away pieces to give to others* as the most poignant emotional/cultural handle. She feels her heart expand with compassion and curiosity to this mixture of kindness, emptiness, and persistent giving! She also resonates with a feeling of fatigue.
2. Elements conveyed: Emily identifies that Joy is conveying:
   A <u>trigger</u> for her emotional distress pattern is seeing others in need.
   <u>Meanings</u>: I have nothing more to give.
   <u>Action tendency</u>: I don't take time to make sure I am ok. I just give and give and give to others in need; even though I am chipping off parts of myself.
3. Missing or vague elements of emotion: Emily is curious to evoke more about how Joy is experiencing this pattern in her body and also her awareness of how this is impacting her.

Emily's Evocative Responses to Invite Elaboration

First she reflects the trigger, the action tendency, and some of the bodily response, then evokes more of the bodily impact.

1. <u>Reflection:</u>
   Emily: (Slowly reflecting in proxy voice.) Empty – nothing left to give, yet when people need, even though I don't have to give I chip away pieces of myself. (Then she pauses for the client to feel the impact of her own words and to say more about that experience.)

2. <u>Invitation to expand more on the bodily-felt element of emotion:</u>
   Emily: Empty – nothing left to give. Tell me more about how that feels in your body to give and give when you feel empty, with nothing more to give and yet constantly chipping off parts of you for others.
3. <u>Targeted question to evoke the bodily-felt sense:</u>
   Emily: You feel empty, and, yet when you see others in need you chip away at your pitcher to keep giving more. Yes? And what's happening inside your body just saying that?

Your Strengths and Discoveries about Evocative Questions and Responding

_____

_____

_____

EFIT Evocative Workout 3: Ariel, Expanding a Passing Reference to a Pivotal Moment

Background

Ariel, 30 years old, is in therapy with the goals of grieving past broken relationships with partners and family and learning how to trust herself to make good decisions in relationships. When she was six years old, her father left the family and they have had very little contact since. The contact they have had was intermittent and unpredictable. She has refused contact with him for the past 14 years. Now he has reached out to her, and she feels intensely mixed feelings, mostly fears of getting her hopes up and then having them dashed when he disappears again, which she thinks is very likely.

Client Expression

ARIEL: My dad sent me a message about meeting for lunch and I got some hope that maybe something might be different, but I don't want to get my hopes up that anything will change between us… I guess I always hoped we could have a relationship again. (Tears up and pauses.) It's a big gamble. He is unpredictable, and his actions always leave me wondering, "What is wrong with me?" Especially an event at 16 really made me wonder that but then I said, "No more!" I'm not risking anymore with him. It's just not worth getting together with my dad anymore. It hurts too much. (Tears stop. Voice is firm.)

This client expression has an added twist, that a therapist will not want to miss. There is a pivotal moment alluded to here (a cataclysmic event – sounding like an attachment injury) that needs to be expanded. Something happened at 16 after which she has not seen her father. Even if the therapist does not choose to evoke and expand on this emotional handle at this moment, it will be important to return to it.

Your Inner Process and Attunement

1. Salience for expansion; resonate in your own body: _____

2. Explicit elements of emotion: _____
3. Vague or missing elements of emotion to evoke or specify:_____

Your Evocative Response to Invite Elaboration

1. Repeat emotional/cultural handle: _____
2. Choose one of the following evocative micro-skills or experiment with all three:

   a. reflect and pause to wait for the client to add more to your reflection,
   b. invite the client to say more about the key element you repeated, or
   c. ask a question targeted at a specific element of emotion:

   _____

   _____

   _____

Emily's Inner Process and Attunement
Compare the emotional handles you have noted with the emotional handles Emily jotted down during her session:

– Don't want to get my hopes up.
– I always hoped.
– Tears up and pauses.
– It's a big gamble.
– His actions always leave me wondering, "What is wrong with me?"
– An event at 16 really made me wonder that but then I said, "No more!"
– I'm not risking anymore with him.
– Hurts too much. (Tears stop. Voice firm.)

1. Salience: Emily is struck by Ariel's phrase, "His actions always leave me with wondering what is wrong with me." She is also struck by her tears over the broken relationship with her dad. She resonates with a stab in her chest at Ariel's wondering if her father's treatment means there something is wrong with her and at her deep sadness over the broken relationship.
2. Elements of emotion conveyed:
   Triggers: Recent message from dad; an event at 16 continues to hurt.
   Meanings: He will hurt me again/my hopes will be dashed; it is a high-stakes risk. View of self: Something is wrong with me; view of other: unpredictable and hurtful.
   Body: Tears up at her broken hopes; voice is firm.
   Conflicting action tendencies: Don't get my hopes up, always hoped, not risking anymore; Questions own worth. Stops her tears. Firmly says will not risk with him again.
3. Missing or vague elements: Ariel's core fear of dad's responses remains vague. Emily is curious to evoke more about the risk and the hurt Ariel feels. The specific event at 16 is missing.

Emily's Evocative Responses

1. <u>Reflection:</u>
   Emily: <u>(Reflecting slowly to invite more.)</u> It's a big gamble to hope; too big a gamble…so many broken hopes. (Then she pauses for Ariel to add more.)
2. <u>Invitation to expand:</u>
   Emily: An event happened when you were 16 that broke your heart, yes? Say more about that.
3. <u>Targeted question</u> to evoke more specificity of her core, underlying fear:
   Emily: Can you say more about the huge risk of getting together with him?

Your Strengths and Discoveries about Evocative Responding

_____

_____

_____

More EFIT evocative workouts are available in the online support material (at routledge. com/9781032151311).

VALIDATION

A validation is an explicit reflection of *what is*, to *give legitimacy* to an emotional experience that is difficult, unacceptable, or even dangerous for clients to experience. Partners may have very different experiences and the EFT therapist finds a way to validate each one's experience. Responses and perspectives that clients are likely to be critical of are framed as valid and understandable. Validating responses convey to partners that different perspectives, emotions, and responses can co-exist in a relationship where persons matter to one another. Validations can be used to contain escalation by making *emotional sense* of differences and validating that each one's experience is valid from their perspective. Validating stuckness opens doors toward exploring, assembling emotion, and discovering new meanings and new action tendencies. It can be very challenging for therapists to accurately name the stuck point. It is difficult to trust the process of assembling emotion and facilitating interpersonal sharing without offering a solution. By virtue of making a current struggle explicit and acceptable to feel, it makes it seem more real, specific, and tangible, and thus, more amenable to change.

Goals of Validations

To calmly and explicitly name conflicting perspectives, emotional experiences, values, longings, action tendencies, or stuck places as both being valid.
To explicitly name felt experience in conflict with expectations from self, others, or the broader social context.
To concretely name both *what their experience is* and what the client feels *it should be* or *is told it should be.*
To validate both the positive intention and the problematic consequences of action tendencies.

How to Form an EFCT Validation

1. Attune to the most poignant dilemma, struggle, stuck place, or conflicting emotional experiences or perspectives.
2. Find words to name this conflict or struggle, linking the elements.
3. Form a validation, by making the struggle explicit and understandable.

EFCT Validation Workouts

EFCT Validation Workout 1: Wayne and Jessica, Validating Positive Intention of an Action Tendency

Context

Wayne is totally committed to being married to Jessica. He has no intention of leaving her but in their typical withdraw-withdraw pattern, he frequently withdraws, and Jessica feels all alone until they reconnect. Although their typical pattern looks like a withdraw/withdraw pattern, Jessica is a more anxious pursuer who withdraws after her attempts to pull Wayne close are unsuccessful.

Client Expression

JESSICA: Sometimes my anger spews out – It's true – I accuse him of all kind of things, that I know send him farther away, when I'm just so afraid he will slip away from me and I'll be all alone again without him!

Your Inner Process and Attunement

1. Attune to the most poignant dilemma, struggle, stuck place, or conflicting emotional experiences or perspectives. _____

_____

2. Find words to name this conflict or struggle, linking/juxtaposing the elements that are in conflict. _____

_____

Your Validation

Form a validation by making the struggle explicit and making *emotional sense* out of the struggle.

_____

_____

After inserting your validation, read it out loud. After this, compare your responses with Emily's below.

Emily's Inner Process and Attunement

1. Emily attunes to Jessica's conflict between her core fear (of Wayne slipping away) and her action tendency (of spewing anger and accusations at him). She feels the dilemma of Jessica doing the very thing that pushes Wayne away; she also feels how Jessica's fears take over and she pushes away the very person she wants to remain close to her. Because this makes sense emotionally, she can name this without feeling judgment or an urgency to get them to change.
2. Emily chooses the words, "so afraid he will slip away" as the core fear motivating Jessica to become accusatory of Wayne and then to see that her words actually do send Wayne into retreating.

Emily's Validation

Emily: It makes sense that if you are so afraid of Wayne slipping away from you, that in your fear, you get louder and push harder to do whatever you can to call him back right away! Your fear takes over and spews out, not as the fear you feel, but as anger against Wayne, pushing him farther and farther away. You don't, yet, have a way to share your fears with him, so that he can stay close and comfort you! Am I getting it? (Adding a tiny seed of an image of a secure attachment bond).

Your Strengths and Discoveries

Compare your inner process and validation response with Emily's. Your response may be very different from hers and that is ok. The important thing is to experiment with being aware of your inner process and attunement and with forming validations. After comparing your response with Emily's, make a note of your strengths to celebrate and/or make a note of what you are discovering from Emily that you want to integrate into your style.

_____

_____

_____

EFCT Validation Workout 2: Reza and Zohreh, Regretting Consequences of an Action Tendency

Context

Reza and Zohreh, first-generation immigrants to Canada from Iran, were high-school sweethearts and have been together for 30 years. The relationship has been tumultuous and also filled with much appreciation for each other. Reza has struggled with anxiety and many self-doubts, throughout his career. Zohreh has supported him and always believed in him.

Client Expression

ZOHREH: I know he needs support and care and I do still care for him but I am getting angry that he's remained stuck, depressed, down on himself all these years! I have tried to convince him he is enough for me, but he's never quite accepted it. I'm exhausted! (Puts her head in her hands and utters a frustrated groan). As much as I hate to admit it, I feel myself pulling away.

Your Inner Process and Attunement

1. Attune to the most poignant dilemma: _____

_____

2. Name this struggle, juxtaposing elements in conflict: _____

_____

Your Validation

Form a validation by making the struggle explicit and making *emotional sense* out of the struggle.

_____

_____

Emily's Inner Process and Attunement

1. Emily attunes to the most poignant dilemma or conflict being that Zohreh loves and cares for Reza but is exhausted and angry and is pulling away from him.
2. Emily finds the words to capture the conflicting elements: Zoreh's action tendency to pull away and her core anger at Reza are in conflict with her love and care for Reza.

Emily's Validation

EMILY: You are exhausted, yes! You have tried for so long to convince him he is your chosen one, and now you are beginning to feel angry with him for never quite believing you. It is very troublesome to notice your frustration rising towards someone you still love but have not ever quite been able to reach!

Your Strengths and Discoveries about Forming Validations

_____

_____

_____

_____

EFCT Validation Workout 3: Katie and Ali, Emotional Threats in a Familiar Pattern

Context

Katie and Ali have an ongoing argument. Ali insists that it is not Katie he is upset with when he walks into a room in disarray or sees toys and books scattered about in their home. "It's me," he insists. "It's all the years as a child when things were out of place and I would get blamed by my parents for making a mess." He describes an immediate knot in his stomach when things are out of place and the immediate feeling of being judged and the urge to escape.

Client Expression

KATIE: He escapes alright! He walks right through the toys straight to the basement! It's his looks that really throw me. When he walks into a messy room, his eyes get wider – kind of glossy – what I call crisp – and his mouth – kind of droops – like a frown, a scowl almost. I see judgement and I feel through and through that he's upset with me, and about to walk away and leave me alone again! And that is precisely what he does!

Your Inner Process and Attunement

1. Attune to the most poignant dilemma: _____

_____

2. Name the struggle, linking elements in conflict: _____

_____

Your Validation

_____

_____

Emily's Inner Process and Attunement

1. Emily's attunement: Emily attunes to two people under attachment threat – Katie sees a look on Ali's face that tells her he is about to walk away from her; Ali sees physical disarray which hits him in the gut with a sense of failure and an impulse to get away.
2. Emily finds these words to formulate the dilemma: What signals a warning to Katie that Ali is about to disappear are the moments Ali is struggling alone with a sense of failure and a need to get away (not from Katie but) from his own bad feelings.

Emily's Validation

EMILY: This makes sense that when a disarray of toys signals to you, Ali, that you have failed and your stomach knots with a sense you are somehow at fault, that you would want to escape from that bad feeling. And of course, Katie when you see that familiar look on his face, just before he does disappear, it makes sense you panic that once again Ali is leaving *you*, because he does walk away in those moments.

Your Strengths and Discoveries about Forming Validations

_____

_____

_____

More EFCT Validation Workouts are available in the online support material (at routledge. com/9781032151311).

EFIT Validation Workouts

The micro-skill of validation is the same skill in EFCT and EFIT but in EFIT the focus of validating is different from validating partners' conflicting perspectives. A validation is an explicit reflection of *what is,* to *give legitimacy* to an emotional experience that is difficult, unacceptable, or even dangerous for clients to have. Validations make feelings, thoughts, and actions that clients may be critical or ashamed of, *acceptable and understandable*, in context. Validations legitimize conflicts between *what clients' current experiences are* and what they feel *they should be or are told they should be.* Validating stuck places and dilemmas can feel counterintuitive to a therapist. It can be challenging to explicitly name a conflict or a dilemma, without offering an immediate solution. It can feel like you are naming, "we are at a dead-end street," without offering a way forward. Trusting the process of emotion, however, identifying clearly where one is, is the starting point to assemble the present-moment experience with more granularity, and in that process, new pathways will open. By virtue of making a current struggle explicit and acceptable to feel, it becomes more real, specific, and tangible, and thus more amenable to exploration and change.

The goals of validations, similar to the goals of validation in EFCT are reviewed here, specifically with individual clients in mind:

> To calmly reflect the explicit existence of perspectives often in conflict, self-protective strategies and actions, emotional experiences, values, longings, stuck places, and needs.
> To explicitly name felt experiences that may be in conflict with expectations from self, others, or the broader social context.
> To concretely name both *what their experience is* and what the client feels *it should be or is told it should be.*
> To validate both the positive intention and the problematic consequences of action tendencies.
> To make it safe for a client to experience painful, difficult experience.

How to Form an EFIT Validation

1. Attune to the most poignant dilemma, struggle, stuck place, or conflicting emotional experiences or perspectives.
2. Find words to name this conflict or struggle, linking or juxtaposing the elements.
3. Form a validation by making the struggle explicit and making "emotional sense" out of the struggle.

EFIT Validation Workout 1: Lola's Internal Battle

Context

Lola is investing in a relationship that is not meeting her needs, with a partner who is uncertain about making a commitment. She keeps hoping for time together and getting let down, over and over. This is reminding her of her past relationships, being with a drug-addicted husband for 20 years and a childhood spent back and forth between a neglectful alcoholic mother and attentive grandparents. She has coped and continues to cope with repeated experiences of getting her hopes up and having them dashed.

Client Expression

LOLA: It's like a battle inside– The Marching Lola says, "Ignore your struggles and just move on; don't stop to complain." And the Boxed Lola is holding so much – stories and songs, tears and rage that have been boxed up and pushed aside all these years.

Your Inner Process and Attunement

1. Attune to the most poignant dilemma, struggle, stuck place, or conflicting emotional experiences or perspectives. _____

   _____

2. Find words to name this conflict or struggle, linking/juxtaposing the elements that are in conflict. _____

   _____

Your Validation

Form a validation by making the struggle explicit and making *emotional sense* out of the struggle

_____

_____

After writing out your validation, read it aloud. After this, compare your responses with Emily's below.

Emily's Inner Process and Attunement

1. Emily attunes to a sense of an internal struggle – of two powerful parts battling to be in charge. She hears how each one part alone would be too much. The Marching Lola would shut everything down (attachment strategy of deactivating) and opening the Boxed Lola (attachment strategy of hyperactivation) would be chaotic!
2. Emily finds these words to validate two strong parts in conflict: marching Lola and Boxed Lola – two good resources, if they can hear from each other and come together as a team.

Emily's Validation

EMILY: You have a clear experience of these two parts in conflict, with both parts giving you important messages. The Marching Lola says, "Keep on going, don't let yourself get discouraged, don't notice how much you are struggling; just keep going." And the Boxed Lola has so many stories, so many emotions, tears and anger, and longings to be seen and listened to, yes?

Your Strengths and Discoveries

Compare your inner process and response with Emily's. Your inner process and response may be very different from hers and that is ok. The important thing is to experiment with being aware of your inner process and attunement and with forming validations. After comparing your response with Emily's, make a note of your strengths to celebrate and/or make a note of what you notice from Emily that you want to integrate into your style.

_____

_____

_____

EFIT Validation Workout 2: Joy, Persevering, Despite Exhaustion

Context

Joy is an African American, Christian woman whom you met in the evocative responding workouts. In a supportive marriage, she works in a human relations job, covering for herself and another manager who is on sick leave. She is open about the pressures she feels as an African American to keep going, to show no signs of struggle or weakness, and to be "the strong Black woman who has no needs of her own." She takes financial responsibility for several family members and invests great care in her employees.

Client Expression

JOY: I am managing okay. (Pauses.) Well, if I stop and notice – truthfully, I am exhausted. I've said before, I am like an empty pitcher – there is no water left, yet I'm pouring, pouring into others' cups, when in fact the pitcher is empty. I keep breaking off parts to give to others. But I cannot stop. Others need. I see their need and my faith and my culture tell me to keep going. It is frustrating.

Your Inner Process and Attunement

1. Attune to the most poignant dilemma: _____

_____

2. Name this struggle, juxtaposing the elements in conflict: _____

_____

Your Validation

_____

_____

Emily's Inner Process and Attunement

1. Emily attunes to Joy's exhaustion with a mixed sense of strong determination and utter fatigue.
2. Emily finds these words to capture the dilemma Joy is facing: compelled by the values from her faith and her culture to keep on giving more and more, yet frustrated and exhausted.

Emily's Validation

EMILY: This truly is a dilemma for you. (Switching to proxy voice.) I am empty, yet my values say, "Keep going, keep giving. Be true to my people. Be true to my faith." At the same time, your body says, "I'm too exhausted to keep doing this but I don't know another way – I don't know what it means to stop and notice something in me is saying I need a rest!"

Your Strengths and Discoveries about Forming Validations

_____

_____

_____

EFIT Validation Workout 3: SuMing, Facing an Impossible Dilemma

Context

SuMing works in the financial sector and immigrated to Canada several years ago, shortly after marrying her high school boyfriend in Hong Kong. She has been working toward making it possible for her husband to come and join her in Canada, and the immigration process is nearly complete. Now she is filled with an enormous dilemma between her marriage commitment and feeling they have grown so far apart that she cannot imagine being intimate with him again or building a life with him in her new country.

Client Expression

SUMING: My core tells me what the right thing is to do but the external distractions are so powerful – they pull me away. I am very conflicted. I want to be true to my core – to my husband back in Hong Kong, who has not yet been able to immigrate to Canada but I am also in love with a fellow in Canada and conflicted about what to do. My core tells me three things: First, I am a good person. Second, I am Chinese and third (voice breaking), I am my parents' child. I am Chinese means I have to stick with things. And I'm a good person means I need to make the right decision and do the right thing. And I am my parent's child means I need to honor my commitments and not bring shame on the family.

Your Inner Process and Attunement

1. Most poignant dilemma: _____

_____

2. Name the struggle, juxtaposing the elements in conflict: _____

_____

Your Validation
Make the struggle explicit and make "emotional sense" of it:_____

_____

_____

Emily's Inner Process and Attunement

1. Emily attunes to this sense of an impossible pull in two directions.
2. She finds the words to capture this dilemma in SuMing's words, "My core tells me what is right – yet I am pulled away."

Emily's Validation

EMILY: (Beginning in proxy voice.) This defines who you are: "I am a good person, I am Chinese, and I am my parents' child. I want to be true to my core and I am in love with a man I am not married to." What a lot of courage it must take to face this dilemma! You don't see the solution yet, but you are facing this difficult dilemma with so much courage and honesty. (Continuing in proxy voice.) "This is me today, conflicted, courageous, and honest!"

Your Strengths and Discoveries about Forming Validations

_____

_____

_____

Another EFIT validation workout is available online (at routledge.com/9781032151311).

HEIGHTENING

Heightening is an important micro-skill in EFT to increase clients' depth of emotional experiencing, an element identified across therapeutic orientations to be the most promising predictor of outcome (Pascual-Leone & Yeryomenko, 2017). In EFT, in particular, the two key elements leading to change, in addition to a secure therapeutic alliance, are depth of emotional experiencing and affiliative interactions (Brubacher & Wiebe, 2019; Greenman & Johnson, 2013). One of the most helpful process guides for attuning to clients' level of experiencing is the Experiencing Scale (EXP; Klein et al., 1969, 1986), developed for research purposes. Therapists familiar with the scale can use it to assess clients' depth of emotional experiencing and their degree of attuning to their inner experience as they explore new meanings, new feelings, and new action impulses. Detail is provided in Chapter 2 of *Stepping into Emotionally Focused Therapy*. An overview of the Experiencing Scale, which follows, is offered to help you focus on emotional depth through the EFCT and EFIT heightening workouts:

- At Levels 1–3, clients are detached from inner experience, giving impersonal, abstract, general, and external descriptions.
- At Level 4, considered the minimum level for experiential therapy, clients are attending to the felt flow of inner experiencing, connecting bodily sensations, meaning-making, and action impulses.
- At Levels 5–7 clients are having expansive emotional experiences that are increasingly concrete, vivid, and alive. Felt shifts and an increasing trust in inner experience emerge as a reliable guide. A fresh way of knowing, new action tendencies, and new meanings evolve.

EFT therapists are constantly seeking to increase clients' capacity to integrate cognitive reflection with affective experience. By orienting clients toward reflecting consciously on their moment-to-moment experience, therapists prime them for shifts in experience, meanings, action tendencies, and resiliency, and for the restructuring of attachment security. Heightening micro-skills are used to savor and deepen awareness of the present moment, emerging emotional experience, new action tendencies and meanings, and personal and interpersonal strengths and resources. Deepening experiencing is an extremely important micro-skill of EFT to slow down and work with present-moment process, in different ways, across all stages of client change.

Therapists heighten with voice tone and with proxy voice (speaking in the first person as though they were the client), with repetitions of images, somatic signals, and clients' words, and by redirecting and repeating clients' core messages. The acronym RISSSSSC, suggesting there is an element of risk with deepened awareness, is how EFT therapists keep these micro-skills in the forefront of their practice. RISSSSSC represents: **R**epetition, **I**mages, **S**imple, **S**oft, **S**low, **S**pecificity, **S**omatic signals, **C**lient's own words. Using the RISSSSSC manner facilitates accessing, savoring, and deepening present-moment emotional experience across all EFT sessions. An EFT therapist continually seeks to balance heightening with containing, so as to engage each client at the optimum emotional *window of tolerance*; that is, to be in touch with, but not overwhelmed by, emotional experience.

If heightening is a micro-skill that is uncomfortable for you, and you are more inclined to rush on quickly, you are not alone. At any point through these micro-skill workouts, you may wish to turn to Part 3 of this book and explore the *reflection workout* on the challenges of *lingering with* and following emotion.

How to Form a Heightening Intervention

1. **Find an emotional handle** (client's words or somatic signs), that strikes you as capturing an emerging or newly distilled emotional experience that you deem valuable to slow down to savor and heighten. This is an important handle to hold and to turn, to open into greater depths and finer, more specific nuances.
2. **Resonate** with the felt sense of this emotional handle and the client's emotional tone in your own body.

3. **Slowly and simply repeat** the emotional handle to open into greater depths, adding *attachment frame* and *specificity* where possible. Match and then heighten clients' emotional tone, varying vocal intonation. Maintain safety with prosody, melodic soothing, simple, soft, slow, and low tone; however, when core emotion requires a more solid, firm intensity, with core anger, for example, is it important to match the client's emotional tone.

EFCT Heightening Workouts

EFCT Heightening Workout 1: Jimmy and Sandy, Fear of Abandonment

Context

A white hetero cisgender couple, Jimmy is an anxious pursuer and Sandy is a withdrawer who lives with an ongoing sense of failure, and a negative sense of self. Jimmy's childhood was marked by his mother being mostly absent due to multiple hospitalizations and losing her to suicide at the age of 9. He typically becomes very critical of Sandy when she spends time playing the piano or going to the gym. He gets very agitated about any clutter or unfinished tasks she leaves behind her and accuses her of going off without him. Her withdrawal to the piano or the gym is frequently triggered by a look of disapproval from Jimmy, so understandably her withdrawal feels like abandonment to him.

Client Expression

JIMMY: (Speaking hesitantly, with broken speech) When Sandy is not there, I am totally alone. (Long pause.) It is not totally logical. I know she will come back, but the aloneness is (another long pause) like when my mother died: When you bury someone, and you know – (speaking very slowly) that they're not –ever going to be – with you – again in your life.

Your Inner Process and Attunement

1. What emotional handle, image, client words, or bodily response strikes you as capturing the most significant marker of emerging or newly distilled emotional experience to savor and heighten? _____

2. How do you resonate in your body? What is your felt sense of this emotional experience?

_____

Your Heightening Response

Combine the words and your felt sense of attachment threat into a heightening response, using elements of RISSSSSC: Slowly and simply repeat the emotional handle to open into greater depths, adding an *attachment frame* and specificity where possible. Match, and then heighten clients' emotional tone, varying your vocal intonation. Maintain safety with prosody, melodic soothing simple, soft, slow, and low tones.

_____

After inserting your heightening response, read it out loud. The tone and pace of *how* a heightening response is said are very important. Hear your own voice saying the words out loud, slowly, simply and either softly or in a tone that matches the client's emotional tone you are wanting to heighten. Experiment with repetition and proxy voice. After this, compare your responses with Emily's below.

Emily's Inner Process and Attunement

1. Emotional handle: What strikes Emily as salient is Jimmy's words, "You bury someone and you know they're not ever going to be with you again in your life."
2. Emily's resonance: Emily has goosebumps as she resonates with the client's words, expressed hesitantly, with many pauses, "You bury someone and you know – that they're not – ever going to be – with you – again." She imagines the sheer attachment panic of this man as a young boy – feeling totally alone – and how that panic is also how he feels in his relationship, when his partner cannot be found.

As she resonates, Emily combines:

1. her goosebumps of attachment anguish (her bodily-felt sense)
2. the client's poignant words "never going to be with you again" and an image of a young boy at his mother's grave
3. the aloneness Jimmy feels in his marriage:

Emily's Heightening Response

EMILY: So alone in your marriage when you cannot find Sandy – aching as much as that young little-boy self all alone at your mother's grave – knowing she's never going to be with you again! So alone without your partner! When Sandy is out of sight and you feel all alone it is a very, very dreadful sense to not know how to bring her back!

Your Strengths and Discoveries
Compare your inner process and heightening response with Emily's. Your response may be very different from hers and that is ok. The important thing is to experiment with being aware of your inner process and attunement and with forming heightening responses. After comparing your response with Emily's, make a note of your strengths to celebrate and/or make a note of what you notice from Emily that you want to integrate into your style.

EFCT Heightening Workout 2: Jack and Karen, Fear of Triggering Depression

Context

A biracial, heterosexual, cisgender couple, in their mid-forties, Jack and Karen are struggling valiantly with many family needs and current job stressors. Jack is successfully getting established in his own flooring business and Karen is studying to upgrade her skills to become a dental assistant. They are very supportive of each other. Their typical pursue/withdraw pattern takes over at times. Karen persists in asking Jack to open up more to her and to lean on her with his troubles. He is very reluctant to do so, however, fearing he may trigger her into depression. A few years earlier she had a long depressive episode, where she was mostly bedridden and reliant upon Jack's care of her and the household, and he continues to try to do all he can for her and to be very self-reliant.

Client Expression

JACK: It's always in the back of my mind. I mean, because I care about and love her and I – I don't <u>ever</u> want that to happen again. (Very emphatic, forceful voice.) I guess I am afraid of her slipping back. So, I just feel the more I can do, the easier it will be on her. (His face suddenly falls, and a very sad look crosses his face.) Just seeing her cry and not want to get out of bed. I mean, it was a very bad time in our life. So, I just feel like the more I can help, you know, it can never go back to that again.

Your Inner Process and Attunement

1. Most significant marker of emerging or newly distilled emotional experience to heighten:

_____

2. Your bodily resonance/felt sense: _____

_____

Your Heightening Response

_____

_____

_____

Emily's Inner Process and Attunement

1. Salient emotional handle: Frightening image of Karen not wanting to get out of bed triggering Jack's determination expressed as, "Don't let it happen again – so the more I can help, the better." What strikes Emily as most prominent is Jack's action tendency of working extra hard to protect Karen from the danger of her depression and how this danger is in the back of his mind all the time!
2. Bodily resonance: Emily feels a weight in her heart – most prominent is Jack's pressure to do all he can to keep the woman he loves from depression, mixed with his fear of her slipping back, and grief at the image of seeing her crying and not wanting to get out of bed.

Emily's Heightening Response
  Read Emily's heightening response out loud in a soft, slow manner, to feel its full impact.

EMILY: Always in the back of your mind – work extra hard to do all you can to keep depression away…so sad and frightening to remember how hard it was (*for both of you*) and you are doing all you can each day, not to burden her, yes?

Note: Emily added a little conjecture that the time of Karen's depression was hard for both of them. She is not sure Jack is ready to acknowledge yet that it was hard for him, but she is seeding the possibility for him to also share more about his experience with Karen.

Your Strengths and Discoveries about Heightening

_____

_____

_____

EFCT Heightening Workout 3: Rona and Anchetta, A Corrective Emotional Experience During a Flashback

Context
Rona and Anchetta are a lesbian couple with a complex pattern. Rona is very affect-avoidant; she survived childhood traumas from punitive parents and sexual abuse by a stranger. Anchetta, also a trauma survivor, likely living with ASD and ADHD, but not interested in being diagnosed, is very demanding of closeness, and highly anxious.

Rona, the more withdrawn partner craves isolation when she is upset and claims that, "Touch is not for me." This is very triggering for Anchetta who, when she feels isolated and alone, becomes desperate and aggressive in her demands. She panics that Rona is not fighting for the relationship. Her gut clenches – and she feels doomed to permanent aloneness. Rona insists she never wants to abandon Anchetta, but that she gets overwhelmed and, "Everything in me pulls me away."

In this particular session, Rona discloses to Anchetta in an encounter, "When the flashbacks come – I don't want anyone near me. It's too dark and cold and scary."

That degree of open, direct sharing with Anchetta is new and touches Anchetta very deeply.

Soon after that, in session, Anchetta notices Rona beginning to have a flashback and she says, "I see it coming. I'm here. You're ok. I don't need to push you. I'm still here."

With the therapist's gentle guidance, to ground Rona in the present, inviting Rona to take a few peaks at Anchetta, Rona has her first flashback without totally dissociating and pulling away from Anchetta.

Client Expression

RONA: That was the first time I felt the cold and dark coming for me – and I wasn't all alone. I trusted your patience with me. That was totally new for me! To be in that cold, dark place of terror and let myself notice you were there with me! I even let you put your foot against my leg. (Rona smiles.) It was comforting.

Your task: Heighten Rona's new emotional experience of the gentle, non-pushy presence of Ancehetta during her most vulnerable state.

Your Inner Process and Attunement

1. Most significant marker of emerging or newly distilled emotion to heighten: _____

_____

2. Your bodily resonance/felt sense: _____

_____

Your Heightening Response

_____

_____

_____

After inserting your heightening response, read it out loud.

Emily's Inner Process and Attunement

1. Salient emotional handle (client's words or somatic signs): *First time in the cold and dark and you were there with me.* This is new for Rona: It was the first time she was not alone in the cold and dark, during a flashback. It was possible and safe to feel Anchetta close by.
2. Resonating with the felt sense of this emotional handle and the client's emotional tone in her own body, Emily feels relief from this new experience. Emily feels an expansiveness opening in her own heart as she sees the vulnerable, terrified Rona, courageously taking a few peaks at Anchetta and welcoming Anchetta's gentle offering of touch with her foot.

Emily's Heightening Response
   Read Emily's heightening response out loud in a soft, slow manner, to feel its full impact.

EMILY: So new – to safely glance at Anchetta and see her patiently sitting there next to you – not pushing, just there for you. So new – to have the courage to glance at her patient face and notice you were not alone. So very, very new – to have a flashback and not be alone in the scary, cold, and dark, but to see and feel Anchetta with you.

Your Strengths and Discoveries about Heightening

_____

_____

_____

EFIT Heightening Workouts

If you are starting with the EFIT Heightening workouts, be sure to review the introduction to the micro-skill of heightening that precedes the EFCT heightening workouts.

EFIT Heightening Workout 1: Fritz, Minimizing Experience

Context

Fritz is processing a random attack he survived decades earlier. He has blocked it out as best he could in his best attempts to minimize the impact of the incident and to ignore the anger and the hatred he feels about it. Recently, however, as he watches the news and the degree of injustice against innocent people across the globe, he finds this incident is troubling him more and more. He struggles with his reactions, feeling he has no right to focus on himself when others are suffering so much more than he is today. "Was it really that bad?" he keeps asking himself.

Client Expression

Read the client's expression below out loud as though you were the client. Then follow the prompts to insert your inner process and attunement and to create your own heightening response.

FRITZ: (Describing what he sees as he recalls seeing himself in the scene of suddenly being attacked from behind.) I see myself with those gangsters kicking me, nothing to grab, nothing to hold on to. (Clenching his fists as he speaks.) It wasn't right!

Your Inner Process and Attunement

1. What emotional handle, image, client words, or bodily response strikes you as capturing the most significant marker of emerging or newly distilled emotional experience for this client who is struggling with his right to recall how this event hurt him? _____

   _____

2. How do you resonate in your body? What is your felt sense of this emotional experience?

   _____

Your Heightening Response

Combine the words and your felt sense of attachment threat into a heightening response, while maintaining safety, using elements of RISSSSSC. Slowly and simply repeat the emotional handle to open into greater depths, adding an *attachment frame* and specificity where possible. Repeat a salient image that captures any newly emerging element of emotion. Match, and then heighten clients' emotional tone, varying vocal intonation. This is likely to evoke a slightly deeper level of experiencing in the client. Maintain safety with prosody, melodic soothing, simple, soft, slow, and low tones.

After inserting your heightening response, read it out loud. The tone and pace of *how* a heightening response is said are very important. Hear your own voice saying the words out loud, slowly, simply, and either softly or in a tone that matches the client's emotional tone that you want to heighten. After this, compare your response with Emily's suggestion below.

Emily's Inner Process and Attunement

1. Salient emotional handle: Client's words that stand out to Emily are the attachment-threatening image of *nowhere to grab, nothing to hold onto* in this dire moment of life-threatening need.
2. Emily finds herself resonating especially with the client's poignant image of attachment panic: *in need of protection, under threat, and totally alone with no one to hold onto.* She feels tension in her own chest with this panicky, desperate sense of sheer isolation when in danger, and she feels confidence in the strength of what appears to be core anger in Fritz's clenching fist, as he says, "It wasn't right!".

Emily's Heightening Response

Read Emily's heightening response out loud in a slow, firm tone, repeating her attachment-panic image and imagining her clenched fist and firm words as she conveys the certainty of his words, "It wasn't right!"

EMILY: (Slowly, with a steady pace.) You ask, "Was my experience really that bad that it should still bother me?" yet you describe it as having been life threatening and terrifying! "Nothing to hold on to. Desperately alone with no one to hold on to!" (Clenching her own fist.) You clench your fists as you say, "Nothing to hold on to!" Terrifying to be all alone with no-one while you felt threatened for your life. Your clenching fists gives power to your words, "It wasn't right!"

Your Strengths and Discoveries

Compare your inner process and response with Emily's. Your responses may be very different from hers and that is ok. The important thing is to experiment with being aware of your inner process and attunement and with forming heightening responses. After comparing your response with Emily's, make a note of your strengths to celebrate and/or make a note of what you notice from Emily that you may want to integrate into your style.

_____

_____

_____

EFIT Heightening Workout 2 with Ivan, Catching an Image as It Flies By

Context

Ivan, an immigrant to North America, speaks rapidly about many changes in his life, jumping quickly from one topic to another. He talks of feeling lost and unable to focus on studying or applying for a new job.

Client Expression

IVAN: (Faltering speech with irregular pacing.) I just cannot focus on anything. I was doing great. I was studying. And then after my dad passed away, I became a ghost. I'm just a ghost that goes everywhere. He does everything... the things he has to do, you know. Studying, preparing for a new job but it's overwhelming. I finished my course, but I'm not really satisfied because I could…I could study better. And…ah…now I'm looking for a job but, in the meanwhile, I have to study too to get prepared for the interviews…. And I can't focus!

Your Inner Process and Attunement

1. Most significant marker of emerging or newly distilled emotions to heighten: _____

_____

2. Your bodily resonance/felt sense: _____

_____

Your Heightening Response

_____

_____

_____

Emily's Inner Process and Attunement

1. Salient emotion handle: Although Ivan rushes by these words, Emily hears a salient emotional handle in his words, "My dad passed away and then I *became a ghost*."
2. Emily resonates with calmness in her own body. In the midst of the client's flurry of words, difficulty focusing, and hurrying from topic to topic, she has identified something that seems to be a clear, understandable trigger for Ivan's scatteredness and inability to focus (action tendencies): His father's passing. Since then, he has felt like a ghost. In her resonance, Emily combines:

    a. Her own body calming down at Ivan's words – *after my dad died – I was a ghost*.
    b. The client's clear statement of trigger – *father died* and the immediate impact – *I became a ghost*.
    c. Becoming a ghost with the loss of his father seems to be a poignant image of the link between the trigger (his father's death) and the disorienting, overwhelming impact that this loss of an attachment figure is having on him.

Emily's Heightening Response
   Read it out loud in a soft, slow manner, to feel its full impact:

EMILY: You are speaking quickly and I'm struck with your words, "My dad passed away and I became a ghost." Going through the motions, going everywhere, doing what you need to do, but since he died it is very difficult to focus. Inside you feel like a ghost since your dad is gone, yes? An emptiness, a disorientation, like "Who am I now," yes?

Your Strengths and Discoveries about Heightening

_____

EFIT Heightening Workout 3: Heightening Core Emotion for Focus

Context

The same client, Ivan, from the previous heightening workout, is an immigrant, facing the recent death of his father in his home country. While fretting over his inability to focus and on being overwhelmed and scattered, tears, core emotion, and disbelief emerge.

Client Expression

IVAN: I am just so scattered. I cannot focus. I keep doing activities that just overwhelm me more and more instead of calming me. Like I feel it's not fair for me. (Eyes filling with tears; voice breaking.) Like sometimes, when I look at his picture...um...I don't believe it. I say, "Is he really gone?" because... I can't take it. It's just too much.

Your Inner Process and Attunement

1. Most significant marker of emerging or newly distilled emotions to heighten: _____
_____

2. Your bodily resonance/felt sense: _____
_____

Your Heightening Response

_____
_____
_____

Emily's Inner Process and Attunement

1. Salient emotion handle: Emily attunes to Ivan's words, "It's not fair!" while his eyes fill with tears and his voice breaks.
2. Bodily resonance: Emily resonates with a frenzied, scatteredness in her heart as she attunes to Ivan, who for a moment focuses on core anger, in the words, "It is not fair" (that father has passed away), combined with core sadness in his tears and words, "It's just too much." She also resonates with the validity of the coping strategy of doubting, "Is he really gone?" when the loss feels like too much to face.

Emily's Heightening Response

Emily chooses to match and then heighten the spark of core anger in Ivan's statement, "It's not fair," since this core anger is the most focused core feeling emerging.

Emily: (In a slow, steady, firm, soothing tone.) It's too much to face that he's really gone. It is not fair! Amidst all the scattered, frenzy you feel, you say, "It is not fair – not fair that my father has passed away!" And then it feels unreal again and you ask, "Is he really gone?" So difficult to believe. It is just not fair. So unfair that your father has passed away! You were not ready for him to die!

Your Strengths and Discoveries about Heightening

_____

_____

_____

THERAPIST TRANSPARENCY

Therapist transparency or self-disclosure is not a significant EFT micro-intervention, though it does serve several functions. It can be used to create safety; to build alliance (around bond, goals, and task elements of alliance); to intensify resonance with the client; to clarify the therapy process, and to validate, normalize, and evoke more engagement from a client who is minimizing or detaching from their present-moment experience. This micro-skill is always to support and expand the client's process. It is important that all therapist self-disclosure return the focus to the client's experience and not become a moment of focusing on the needs or the struggle of the therapist.

Therapist transparency can involve disclosure about:

1. The therapist's life experiences and social location. For example, "I do not know what it is like to experience exclusion because of the color of my skin, but as an immigrant to this country, I know something of feeling I am not wanted in some circles."
2. The therapist's present-moment emotional experience in the session. For example: "I feel sad as you say…"; "My heart drops as I hear you say…"; "I also have moments of self-doubt and questioning my worth, for example, when…". This transparency can create a powerful moment of validation for clients who have never been validated for their vulnerable emotions.
3. The therapeutic process and how the therapist is working in the moment. When a therapist clearly and confidently describes the therapeutic process, it can help to build or repair the therapeutic alliance. For example, describing *how* delineating the present pattern is part of the path toward repair; *how* the work we are doing just now is directly related to reaching the goals you have set for your therapy; and what it is about encounters that make them both uncomfortable and helpful. Transparency about the therapy process helps to build task alliance and strengthen clients' confidence that the therapy process is relevant to their concerns. The workouts here focus primarily on this final aspect.

How to Formulate the Micro-Skill of Therapist Transparency

1. **Attune:** Identify what strikes you about the therapeutic alliance or the client's need for safety, or support, or trust where your transparency could be of value.

2. **Check your own bodily-felt sense** as you anticipate sharing. Personal disclosure can feel risky, so it is important to take a conscious breath and be mindful of your own presence, while you disclose. (Similar to helping clients anticipate an encounter, in EFT Move 3, there is an element of risk in sharing.)

3. **Disclose** to the client, mentioning how you hope your transparency relates to them or the relationship between you. (Similar to EFT Move 3)

4. **Check for the impact** on them, being certain to retain or return the focus to the client's experience. (Similar to EFT Move 4)

Therapist Transparency Workouts

References are made in the following workouts to therapist transparency and moves of the EFT Tango. If the EFT Tango terminology is unfamiliar to you, you may wish to check Part 2 for a complete introduction to the EFT Tango.

The EFCT Therapist Transparency workout applies to a situation where therapist transparency is used to create or restore safety between partners and within the therapeutic alliance. Transparency about the therapeutic process is combined with the therapist's awareness of their own bodily arousal and therapeutic presence in these challenging moments.

EFCT Therapist Transparency Workout: To Restore Safety with Emmett and Tracy

Context

Emmett, a cisgender Black man and Tracy, a cisgender White woman, have a highly escalated pattern with Emmett withdrawing and defending and Tracy pursuing and criticizing. Emmett describes a very disturbing recent experience of being racially profiled and treated unacceptably in a clothing store. While the therapist was validating Emmett's frustration and the unfair exclusion he experiences, Tracy reacted in a sharp tone to the therapist.

Client Expression

Read the client's expression below out loud. Given the context described above, follow the prompts to identify your inner process and attunement and to form an expression of therapist transparency (self-disclosure) that you feel could help to create safety and be of value to the clients.

TRACY: (To the therapist.) Seems like you are taking his side here! We don't know if it was a racist act. Maybe the cashier was just having a bad day! We just don't know, so I wish he wouldn't get so upset.

Your Inner Process and Attunement

1. Attune: Identify what strikes you about the therapeutic alliance, the need for safety, and how your transparency could be of value. _____

2. Check your own bodily-felt sense as you anticipate sharing. (This is like anticipating an encounter where you are the discloser, so there is an element of risk.) Breathe and be mindful of your own level of arousal and presence. (Similar to Move 3.) _____

_____

Your Therapist Transparency Response

1. **Disclose** to the client: Begin with reflecting on the significant part of the client's message and describe how your disclosure is directly related to them or to the relationship between you. (Similar to Move 3.) _____

_____

_____

2. **Check for the impact** on them. (Similar to Move 4.) _____

_____

After inserting your responses, compare with Emily's below. Take note of similarities and differences, identifying your strengths and anything you might want to consider integrating into your EFT style of using therapist transparency.

Emily's Inner Process and Attunement

1. Attunement: Emily immediately feels a need to create safety and to attend to the alliance and to let the couple know – with transparency – that she will interrupt to maintain or re-establish safety.
2. Body: Emily notices her heart is racing in this very important moment, where Emmett's experience of racial exclusion is being discounted by his wife. She decides her transparency about how she wants to create safety is the most important message for her to deliver at this moment. She is mindful of the importance of her voice. There is no time to breathe deeply but as she begins to speak, she uses a slow voice to get her own balance while also looking directly at one and then the other of the partners in front of her to help her to co-regulate.

Emily's Transparency to Create Safety and Build Task Alliance

EMILY: I know it is difficult for you to see Emmett feeling upset, but I want to assure you that I am trying to understand both of your perspectives and if I sense one of you is unintentionally hurting the other one with your words, I will step in to stop what is happening, like I just did now. (To Tracy): Emmett's experience is that he was treated badly because of the color of his skin. That is indeed totally unacceptable that he should have to endure that experience. I hear it is hard for you to hear that! No doubt you wish it didn't happen. (To Emmett): I want to make it safe for you Emmett to have your experience heard and validated. (To Tracy): And I want to make it possible and safe for you, Tracy, to hear what this man you love is saying and what he experiences out in the world that you and I do not. I want to make it safe for both of you! How does that sound to each of you?

Your Strengths and Discoveries

Compare your inner process and transparency with Emily's. Your responses may be very different from hers and that is ok. The important thing is to experiment with being aware of your inner process and attunement, to reflect on what you have to disclose to the client about yourself or about your activity in the therapy process that could move their therapy forward, and to then form a genuine self-disclosure or expression of therapist transparency. Note your strengths to celebrate and/or what you notice from Emily that you want to integrate into your style.

_____

_____

_____

A second EFCT transparency workout is available in the online support material (at routledge.com/9781032151311).

EFIT Therapist Transparency Workout: Transparency about the Therapy Process with Max

This EFIT therapist transparency workout employs therapist transparency about the therapeutic process, to be clear with the client about their intentions in the moment, to maintain safety and understanding.

Context

From the first session of therapy, Max, first introduced in an empathic attunement workout, indicated he has a big fear that has been stalking him for nearly 20 years. The fear is of consciously remembering the dead body of his friend for whose death he is responsible. He spent time in jail for criminal negligence causing death, for being the driver in a street racing crash that took his friend's life and left him badly damaged. "It was the race from hell," he says.

> I know how badly my body was damaged and I know I was walking around, after the accident, so in the back of my mind, after all these years is this fear that I will recall how bad Léo looked. For some reason, this terrifies me.

In therapy, Max has had various encounters with an imaginal Léo as he remembers him when he was still alive. They have told each other they love one another; he has experienced an imaginal Léo telling him that he is fully forgiven for his death. His guilt has receded, and he has expressed remorse and responsibility to an imaginal Léo. The therapist is aware, however, that together they have not explicitly entered the scene of the accident and looked down at the ground to Léo's body. The therapist recognizes that they also feel some of the terror that they sense Max feels about seeing his friend's body at the scene of the accident. They realize that they have been postponing something that needs to be done and that is likely tolerable now for Max.

Your task: As a therapist, you hear the client has stabilized from an encounter with an image of his friend as he remembered him in real life. You also know you have not yet gathered the courage or felt he was ready to face an image of the person he is fearful of seeing. It would be easy to let it go, but if you are honest with yourself, you feel his fear is still alive and therefore needs to be revisited. How could you use transparency about the therapy process to share with Max how you feel it is important to return to explore what he has identified as his biggest fear and to shape an encounter with the body he fears seeing?

Client Expression

MAX: This fear of having a conscious memory of seeing Léo's body at the accident doesn't come up as much as it used to, but it's just – it's something that's kind of – it's always been there at the back of my head, right? But it's so much better with the work we already did – speaking to Léo as I remember him before the accident and sensing his forgiveness helped a lot. But yeah, I'd have to say the fear is still always there…

Your Inner Process and Attunement

1. Attune: Identify what strikes you about the therapeutic alliance or the client's need for safety, or support, and how your transparency could be of value. _____

_____

2. Check your own bodily-felt sense as you anticipate sharing. (This is like anticipating an encounter where you are the discloser, so there is an element of risk.) Breathe and be mindful of your own level of arousal and presence. (Similar to Move 3) _____

_____

Your Therapist Transparency

1. **Disclose** to the client: Begin with reflecting on the significant part of the client's message and describe how your disclosure is directly related to them or the relationship between you. (Similar to Move 3) _____

_____

_____

_____

2. **Check for the impact** on him. (Similar to Move 4) _____

_____

Emily's Inner Process and Attunement

1. Attunement: Emily is aware that she has not yet helped him to face his biggest fear of seeing Léo at the scene of his death. She initially invited Max to do an imaginal encounter with Léo as he remembered him alive, in order to not overwhelm him and to slice this very scary process in thin slices to keep it safe. However, she hears that recalling seeing the body in the actual scene is what terrifies him. She senses her honesty about this process could convey respect and clarity and help ease her into shaping this one more transformative encounter with Léo's body in a safe and transformative way.
2. Therapist's bodily sense: Emily checks her **own bodily-felt sense** as she anticipates sharing with Max. (She feels the element of risk in inviting Max to do the very thing he fears; She takes a conscious breath and decides that it will further regulate her and help her to help Max do what he needs to do if she is transparent about her process.)

Emily's Transparency

EMILY: You still fear the fear every day of seeing Léo's body at the scene of the accident. You've had several encounters with the imaginal Léo as you remember him alive, but we have not yet looked directly at the Léo at the accident. I felt like we walked close to the edge of this danger you fear but I'm not sure I have helped you fully face it. I would feel I was doing you a disservice if we left that fear in the background and didn't visit it more fully. Does that make sense? I hear how much safety you have gained – how experiencing an image of Léo forgiving you for his death has helped a lot – and yet the fear of recalling how he looked still haunts you. I want to help you walk back into the scene of the accident in a way that is safe for you – to approach that image of Léo's body. (Similar to the anticipation part of shaping an encounter, in Move 3, as detailed in Part 2.)

To check for the impact of this disclosure on Max, Emily adds: How does that sound to you? (Similar to Processing an encounter, in Move 4 as detailed in Part 2.)

   Your strengths and discoveries about what you have to disclose to a client about yourself to move their therapy forward.

_____

_____

_____

   A second EFIT transparency workout is available in the online support material (at routledge.com/9781032151311).

EMPATHIC CONJECTURES

Empathic conjectures are tentatively offered reflections that go slightly beyond the leading edge of what a client has verbalized. EFT therapists seek to help clients discover and safely explore emotions that are "frightening and/or alien and unacceptable" (Bowlby, 1988, p. 139) and lie on the leading edge of awareness. Conjectures could be called *hunches detected through attunement to* attachment themes and to the entire context of what the client has shared, verbally and non-verbally. Made at the leading edge of experience and within an attachment/contextual frame, empathic conjectures expand clients' awareness and articulation of experience. Images, bodily signs, sudden exits, or interruptions are all emotional handles, indicating that a high level of emotional experience is on the leading edge of awareness.

Goal of Empathic Conjectures

The goal of an empathic conjecture is to expand the client's depth of emotional engagement. It is to engage clients more deeply in the emerging edges of their own implicit experience, thus opening new depths and new perspectives. This is what Rice (1974) called *evocative empathy* or *empathy on the leading edge.* The goal is not to offer insight or to explain *why, but rather* to expand each client's emotional experience – their bodily-felt, meaning-making, action process – and their capacity to put words to their newly emerging experience. An indication of the usefulness of an empathic conjecture is when a client responds with some form of, "Exactly – that's it! I just didn't have the words for it!"

To form empathic conjectures, therapists stay very close to clients' experience, yet slightly on the leading edge. They do this by finding an emotional handle or focal point to expand. They are attuned to their own bodily-*felt sensing* of a client's story and to the context of what attachment theory conveys about human needs for connection and safety. The therapist links the explicit message from the client to their hunch of implied emotional experience. When offering conjectures, it is important to convey tentativeness and to take time to check if the communicated understanding accurately matches the client's expanding experience. The therapist's use of proxy voice while offering an empathic conjecture brings the emotional experience alive and gives the client an opportunity to taste the experience and check if it matches their internal experience. As with all empathic reflections, it is paramount that a client perceives that the therapist understands accurately. If a therapist is too far on the leading edge with a conjecture, a client is likely not to recognize that it matches with their experience, or they may agree intellectually but not be engaged with their own emotional experiencing.

This section contains general empathic conjecture workouts. There are also three special types of conjectures included later: *seeding attachment* and *catching bullets* (in Part 1) and *slicing risks thinner* (included in Part 2 of this book with Tango Move 3).

To form an empathic conjecture, listen for verbal hints or bodily signals of emotions that are not expressed directly, while also being intently immersed in the client's words and their larger contextual experience and positions and patterns of interaction. As Martin (2016) says, tune into more than the last few words.

Examples of empathic conjectures at "hints" of emotion on the leading edge:

1. An individual's sudden glance to the floor is explicit, however, the therapist detects a hint of fear or guilt as related to the larger context of the client's experience and offers an empathic conjecture (with tentativeness and in proxy voice):

   I may be off here, but as you suddenly looked to the floor, I am wondering if your familiar *blame me pattern* just showed up. That is, "When something goes wrong, it must be me – what did I do wrong?" Did that just come up for you again?

2. You said, "I don't blame myself for her suicide. She had to do what he had to do" and then your face suddenly dropped and you threw up your hands and looked in my face, almost as if you were saying, "What could I have done?" I wonder, is there, perhaps, an edge of you wondering, "Was there more I could have done?"

The process for forming conjectures that you will have an opportunity to follow in each empathic conjecture workout is below.

How to Form Empathic Conjectures

Your Inner Process and Attunement

1. **Identify explicit and implicit signals that hint at the emotional experience of threat, security, core emotion, or longings on the leading edge:**

Examples:

Verbal hint: "I'm not afraid," might hint at some fear a client is trying not to feel.

Non-verbal hint: A smile, folding arms, twisting fingers or shift in vocal tone or pace indicate that something emotional is happening. A smile or folded arms while a client says, "It doesn't bother me" hints at a different message on the leading edge, such as, "It does bother me.").

2. **Identify relevant context:** Identify what you know about this client's larger context. This could be the cultural context, the relational context, or the context of the client's typical pattern in the face of difficulty or danger, including typical triggers, meanings made, or action tendencies when under threat.

3. **Find words to capture your inference of the leading-edge emotion:** Identify what you hear implied on the leading edge. Resonate with your felt sense of this inference.

Your Empathic Conjecture

1. **With a tentative tone, link** some explicit expression from the client to a thin slice of experience you hear implied. State it simply, experimenting with a proxy voice to help both yourself and your client *experience* these new words about their present-moment emotional experience.

2. **Invite the client to confirm or disconfirm.** In real life, if the client seems emotionally disengaged and simply "agrees," EFT therapists will ask the client *how* the conjecture fits for them or what it captures about their experience.

EFCT Empathic Conjecture Workouts

EFCT Empathic Conjecture Workout 1: Toby and Crystal, Being Careful

Context

Toby, a rather withdrawn partner speaks in carefully measured tones, as though treading very carefully. He wants very much to please his partner, Crystal, and to build a life with her. She pushes him to speak more and to disclose more, making references to the past where his holding back from her resulted in him texting other women. Both partners are confident he doesn't do this anymore. Crystal emphasizes that she trusts that he is "all in" in their relationship now. The more Crystal demands openness, the more Toby tries to give her what she obviously longs for, and the harder he tries, the more frozen he seems to get.

Client Expression

Read the client's expression below out loud as though you were the client(s). Then follow the prompts to insert your inner process and attunement and to create your own empathic conjecture.

TOBY: (With a hurried pace) I am trying not to hold back so much, because I know she wants to hear more from me. But we are both in the middle of so many work-related stressors and I constantly try to do as much as I can, so as not to overload her. I am very careful not to burden her with my problems.

Your Inner Process and Attunement

1. Identify explicit and implicit signals that hint at the emotional experience of threat, security, and longings, on the leading edge:

   Verbal: _____

   Non-verbal: _____

2. Relevant context (what you know about this client's position and pattern and greater socio-cultural context): _____

   _____

3. Find words to capture your inference of the leading-edge emotion: _____

   _____ Resonate with your felt sense of

   this inference. What do you feel? _____

Your Empathic Conjecture

1. With a tentative tone, link some explicit expression from the client to a thin slice of experience you hear implied. Experiment with proxy voice. _____

   _____

2. Invite the client to confirm or disconfirm. _____

After inserting your empathic conjecture read it out loud. Your tone and pace are important. Hear your own voice saying the words out loud, with tentativeness and an invitation to the client to confirm or disconfirm the fit with their experience. After this, compare your responses with Emily's below.

Emily's Inner Process and Attunement

1. Explicit and implicit signals of emotional experience on the leading edge that Emily identifies:
   a. Non-verbal: His hurried pace may imply some sense of pressure and anxiety.
   b. Verbal: "Try not to hold back," implies he is holding back; "very careful not to burden her with my problems," implies a perception she would be burdened with his sharing, thus it feels risky to share; "constantly try to do as much as I can, so as not to overload her," implies a fear of overloading her.
2. Relevant context: Emily identifies that Toby is very careful to get it right with Crystal and that Crystal is pushing him to be more open with her. Although Crystal claims to fully trust that he "is in" she is afraid of his holding back. Crystal's recent depression must still be fresh in Toby's mind and Toby's turning to other women must also be fresh in Crystal's mind.
3. Emily finds these words to capture the leading-edge emotion: Emily infers that Toby is experiencing a difficult dilemma: feeling pressure to share more, while at the same time, fearing overloading Crystal and having no idea of what to share with her.
   Emily resonates with a felt sense of Toby feeling pressure and fear.

Emily's Empathic Conjecture

With a tentative tone, Emily links Toby's careful tone and rapid pace with her hunch of fear and pressure.

EMILY: You speak so carefully as you describe what must feel like a real dilemma. (Continues in proxy voice.) I want to share more, as she asks. I must. I want to make her happy. But oh – oh – too risky! What if I burden her? What is there about me she wants to know? Am I getting the conflict you seem to feel? Pressure to share more and fear of burdening her?

Your Strengths and Discoveries

Compare your inner process and empathic conjecture with Emily's. Your response may be very different from hers and that is ok. The important thing is to experiment with being aware of your inner process and attunement and with forming empathic conjectures with tentativeness, while being open to being corrected if your words do not fit in the moment for the client. After comparing your response with Emily's, make a note of your strengths to celebrate and/or make a note of what you notice from Emily that you want to integrate into your style.

_____

_____

_____

EFCT Empathic Conjecturing Workout 2: Toby and Crystal, Deepening the Fear

Context

Toby and Crystal as above. Toby begins to share more about his fear of opening up as linked to his fear of Crystal falling into depression again.

Client Expression

TOBY: Three years ago, Crystal suffered a major depressive episode. It's always in the back of my mind. I mean, because I care about her and love her and I know I don't <u>ever</u> want her depression to happen again! (Voice is very vigorous) So I just feel the more I can do, the harder I work, the easier it will be on her. (His face suddenly falls – and a very sad look comes over him.)

Your Inner Process and Attunement

1. Identify explicit and implicit signals of threat, security, and longings, on the leading edge:

   a. Verbal: _____

   b. Non-verbal: _____

2. Relevant context: _____

3. Find words for your inference of the leading-edge emotion: _____
_____ Resonate with
your felt sense of this inference. What do you feel?_____

Your Empathic Conjecture

1. With a tentative tone, link some explicit expression to a thin slice of experience you hear implied. Experiment with proxy voice. _____
_____

2. Invite the client to confirm or disconfirm. _____

Emily's Inner Process and Attunement

1. Verbal and non-verbal signals of emotional experience on the leading edge: Emily hears an implication of alive, unexpressed fear on the leading edge of experience in several phrases and several non-verbal signals:
    • his vigorous voice (may imply "Work hard to keep depression away.")
    • "always in the back of my mind" (Implies this fear is stalking him)
    • "I don't <u>ever</u> want that to happen!" (Implies fear of it happening again.)
    • sudden fallen face. (May imply that thoughts of Crystal's depression trigger sad memories, and may also trigger remorse for his past turning to other women.)
2. Relevant information about larger context and position and pattern: Emily considers the significant external work stressors Toby and Crystal are experiencing. Crystal suffered from depression in the past. Toby downregulates his own experience and works very hard to please and help Crystal. Crystal pushes Toby to share more. Toby doesn't want to overload Crystal. Toby's withdrawal in the past included texting other women, though he is not currently doing so.
3. Emily finds words to capture her inference of the leading-edge hint of implied emotion: Fear and caution and pressure to work hard so Crystal's depression does not recur.

Emily's Empathic Conjecture

EMILY: Help me know if I understanding you correctly. (Proxy voice.) Always in the back of my mind, 'Don't ever let her fall into depression again!' I get a sense that you are feeling constantly on guard, like, "I have to get it right with her – I can't slip and make any wrong moves, or she might get depressed again." This sounds very frightening, and it must feel safer just to hold yourself back when you are so fearful of triggering her depression again. Am I understanding?

Your Strengths and Discoveries with Forming an Empathic Conjecture

_____

_____

_____

EFCT Empathic Conjecture Workout 3: Ted and Jed, A Pursuer's Fear on the Leading Edge

Context

Ted and Jed have a volatile pursue/criticize – withdraw/defend pattern. Ted's anxieties frequently come out as angry criticisms toward his partner, Jed, who is very guarded, protecting himself from Ted's next torrent of complaints, sometimes with defense, but mostly with silence and distancing!

Client Expression

TED: The thing is, I would do anything for him, but…. (Eyes filling with tears; pauses, briefly.) The way it goes in our house (continues on speaking rapidly and with an agitated tone; all signs of tears disappear quickly) is that I can spend hours cooking up a fantastic dinner, and…

Your Inner Process and Attunement

1. Identify explicit and implicit signals of threat, security, and longings, on the leading edge:

   a) Verbal: _____
   b) Non-verbal: _____

2. Relevant context: _____
3. Find words for your inference of the leading-edge emotion: _____
   _____ Resonate with
   your felt sense of this inference. What do you feel?_____

Your Empathic Conjecture

1. With a tentative tone, link some explicit expression from the client to a thin slice of experience you hear implied. Experiment with proxy voice. _____

   _____

   _____

2. Invite the client to confirm or disconfirm. _____

Emily's Inner Process and Attunement

1. Signals that hint at the emotional experience of threat, security, and longings, on the leading edge: Emily is struck by the sudden change in Ted's demeanor when he shifts from his eyes filling with tears and his brief pause after saying, "but…" to his suddenly stopping the tears and beginning to speak rapidly about how things go when he cooks up a fantastic dinner.
2. Relevant information about larger context and position and pattern: Given their repetitive pattern of the more Ted complains and pushes, the more Jed withdraws and protects himself, she hears in Ted's tears and "but" an implied threatening message that Jed is perhaps not as committed as Ted is to their relationship.

3. Emily finds these words to capture the leading-edge emotion: Underlying fear and sadness that Jed may not be committed to him as he is to Jed.

Emily's Empathic Conjecture

EMILY: Can we just slow down a moment, please? You said you would do anything for Jed, but…and your eyes filled with tears – almost like all those tears had more to say before you switched them off and began speaking rapidly about cooking dinner. It almost felt as though you were saying, "I would do anything for him, but – but I'm not sure he would do the same for me, am I hearing you correctly?"

Your Strengths and Discoveries about Forming Empathic Conjectures

_____

_____

_____

Find more EFCT Empathic Conjectures online (at routledge.com/9781032151311).

EFIT Empathic Conjecture Workouts

If you have come directly to the EFIT workouts in empathic conjectures, please read the goals, functions, and process of forming this micro-skill as it is introduced as a lead-in to the EFCT empathic conjecture workouts. As you begin these workouts, keep in mind that you are moving slightly beyond the leading edge of what a client has verbalized, based on what you have picked up from their larger story. Practice in identifying frightening, alien, and/or unacceptable emotion that lies on the leading edge of awareness will help you to engage clients more deeply in the emerging edges of their own implicit experience, thus opening new depths and new possibilities.

EFIT Empathic Conjecture Workout 1 with Mona: Weighted Down in Depression and Grief

Context

Mona, 25 years old, identifies as an Indigenous woman of color, begins therapy in a lethargic state, very depressed, finding it difficult to get out of bed most days. She openly acknowledges that her closest confidant all her life was her mother. She stayed home a lot and rarely engaged with friends. Her strategy for regulating emotion is to suppress her experience into one of numbness and quiet. This pattern, one she has used for most of her life, has been accentuated in the past few years following the sudden death of her mother, who died tragically in an accident where she was hit by an oncoming bus.

In her first sessions of therapy, Mona and the therapist find some coherence through identifying her pattern and assembling her emotional experience. Gradually, she can identify a bodily sense of emptiness and feel some stirring of pain in that emptiness, feeling physically weighted down. She discovers an attribution she makes that "part of me is missing." She is owning her typical action tendency of basic avoidance and withdrawing from others, to cope with loss. This assembling of emotions begins to bring order to her experience which at first, she said was "difficult to explain." The coherence she arrives at with her therapist is that to avoid feeling the pain of missing her mom, she avoids her own emotions, and she avoids reaching out to anyone else for comfort. In this coherence, she is beginning to feel the twinges of the pain of her loss.

Client Expression

MONA: I don't want to blame her for getting hit by that bus. It wasn't her fault. I don't want to be angry at her for dying. But here I am, three years since she died, totally lethargic and depressed. Mostly numb, nothing makes me happy. Not even my adorable baby nephew. I don't really feel sad either. But some days, I can barely get out of bed. (Voice tone is very flat.)

Your Inner Process and Attunement

1. Identify explicit and implicit signals that hint at emotional experience of threat, security, and longings, on the leading edge:

   a. Verbal: _____

   b. Non-verbal: _____

2. Relevant context (what you know about this client's position and pattern and greater socio-cultural context): _____

3. Find words to capture your inference of the leading-edge emotion: _____
_____ Resonate with your felt sense of
this inference. What do you feel?_____

Your Empathic Conjecture

1. With a tentative tone, link some explicit expression from the client to a thin slice of experience you hear implied. Experiment with proxy voice. _____

_____

2. Invite the client to confirm or disconfirm. _____

Emily's Inner Process and Attunement

1. Signals that hint at emotional experience on the leading edge: Emily identifies

   a. Verbal: "I don't want to blame my mom," implies a part of her does blame her but doesn't want to. Her words, "I don't want to be angry at her for getting hit by that bus," and "I don't want to blame her for dying," imply that perhaps a part of her is angry at her mom for getting hit and dying.

   b. Non-verbal: Her flat tone sounds to Emily almost like Mona is holding back from feeling anything, and especially from the anger she mentions not wanting to feel.

2. Relevant context: Emily identifies that this unexpected loss of her mother, when Mona already had a pattern of downregulating and not reaching out to others has literally frozen her world. It

is as though her world has come to a standstill. Emily also recognizes how anger is a life-giving part of emotional pain.

3. Leading-edge emotion: Emily finds these words to capture her inference of the leading-edge emotion: Mona seems to be holding back a lot of legitimate anger for how her world was suddenly and unexpectedly frozen and forever altered.

   Emily resonates with a felt sense of holding back; holding back to keep from exploding in tears or rage!

Emily's Empathic Conjecture

With a tentative tone, Emily links Mona's comments about not wanting to be angry to her bodily-felt sense of numbness and her sense that Mona is holding back a lot of legitimate anger for how her world was suddenly and unexpectedly changed forever.

EMILY: I hear you saying, "I don't want to blame my mom. I don't want to be angry at her for suddenly disappearing and changing my life forever." (continuing in proxy voice) "Hold back, don't feel, it's all too much, so hold it all back." Yet I sense, and I could be wrong, that you are understandably somewhat angry with her, yes? Just maybe you say, "Why weren't you more careful? Why did you end up leaving us?" Something like that? I sense you are working so hard to hold all that back! Am I getting how it is for you?

Your Strengths and Discoveries

Compare your inner process and empathic conjecture with Emily's. Your response may be very different from hers and that is ok. The important thing is to experiment with being aware of your inner process and attunement and with forming empathic conjectures with tentativeness, while being open to being corrected if your words do not fit in the moment for the client. After comparing your response with Emily's, make a note of your strengths to celebrate and/or make a note of what you notice from Emily that you want to integrate into your style.

_____

_____

_____

EFIT Empathic Conjecture Workout 2 with Maryam: Confusion May Contain Hope

Context

Maryam is an immigrant from a patriarchal society, without a secure social support network in her new country. Her new husband whom she immigrated with has just filed for divorce and her main supports, her father in particular, are still in Egypt.

Client Expression

MARYAM: I feel my dad is pulling for me to come back home (voice quivers), but I really want to make it here (voice growing strong), in my new country. I hear him wanting me to be successful, but I also feel he is pulling me back. I don't see him picturing me being a very independent woman. (Pause.) I don't know. (Quizzical look on her face; pauses.) Whenever I was used to tell him that I can handle my life, his face was always full of doubts, as though he did not believe me. The love is there. I know that he's very concerned about me and he wants me to be strong and successful. He wants me to be independent. But I feel he still sees me as his little daughter (smiling through tears) as a 6-year-old girl. He still loves me the way that he used to back then. But I need to know he, or at least someone, believes I can make it in this new country.

Your Inner Process and Attunement

1. Identify explicit and implicit signals of threat, security, and longings, on the leading edge:

   a. Verbal: _____

   b. Non-verbal: _____
2. Relevant context: _____
3. Find words to capture your inference of the leading-edge emotion: _____ _____ Resonate with your felt sense of this inference. What do you feel?_____

Your Empathic Conjecture

1. With a tentative tone, link some explicit expression from the client to a thin slice of experience you hear implied. Experiment with proxy voice. _____

   _____
2. Invite the client to confirm or disconfirm. _____

Emily's Inner Process and Attunement

1. Signals that hint at emotional experience on the leading edge: Emily identifies:

   a. Verbal: Dad is pulling me back; he loves me; doubts if I can be successful on my own; wants me to be successful; sees me as a six-year-old.
   b. Non-verbal: tears; voice strengthens at points and quivers at other times; quizzical look after she says her dad doesn't see her as an independent woman, after which she added, "I don't know."
2. Relevant context: Emily identifies her sense of isolation as an immigrant, the grief of her husband's sudden departure, and the pull she feels toward her family. She hears the theme of a patriarchal culture's importance of a man believing in her.
3. Leading-edge emotion: Emily resonates with a felt sense of "good confusion" in that Maryam has lots of tears and smiles when she speaks of her father seeing her as a six-year-old. Most striking is the look of puzzlement when she says, "He doesn't see me as an independent woman," followed by her pause as she said, "I don't know.'

Emily's Empathic Conjecture

With a tentative tone, Emily links some explicit expressions from the client to a thin slice of experience she hears implied. (Proxy voice.)

EMILY: You are feeling the pain of your husband leaving you and now the pain of feeling that in your father's eyes, you are still a child whom he may not believe can make it on her own. "Who believes in me today," you are wondering, yes? Almost like you are saying, "Who can I rely on to say, 'You can do this!'" I am struck with your pause when you said, "My father doesn't see me as an independent woman," and then you stopped and said, "I don't know" with a very puzzled look on your face. Almost as though you were saying, "Or does he? Just perhaps he knows I can make it here. Just perhaps he knows I have what it takes to rebuild my life here, with all the love coming from him and the entire family." Am I hearing you correctly? Is that what your look of confusion is saying, when you said, "I don't know"? Just maybe he does believe you can do this?

Your Strengths and Discoveries about Forming Empathic Conjectures

_____

_____

_____

EFIT Empathic Conjecture Workout 3 with Fritz: Injustice But Don't Feel the Rage

Context

Fritz, whom you met in the heightening workout, struggles to feel he has a right to process his decades-old trauma when people are suffering the world over! He copes by trying to rationalize how this happened and is determined not to allow the trauma to make him a vengeful person. However, he is beginning to feel the impact of this unprocessed trauma which he has never explored.

Client Expression

FRITZ: Actually, this incident is having repercussions in my daily life. (Speaking in a matter-of-fact voice, in a reporting manner.) They are not negative but intense. And they are impacting me, in intense ways. There is pain and injustice. Because it happened out of the blue. It happened in a very severe way. (Jaw tenses.) I nearly died. I never really understood why. These *questions still linger on my soul* and I try to understand them, but you know, sometimes it is very hard to do that. And I suspect, it comes out in other ways. Like in my outbursts of rage. But I do not want to be an angry man. I am trying to understand why this happened!

Your Inner Process and Attunement

1. Identify explicit and implicit signals on the leading edge:

   a. Verbal: _____

   b. Non-verbal: _____

2. Relevant context (client's position, pattern, and socio-cultural context): _____

_____

3. Words to capture your inference of the leading-edge emotion: _____
_____ Resonate with your felt sense of this
inference. What do you feel?_____

Your Empathic Conjecture

1. With a tentative tone and proxy voice. _____

_____

2. Invite the client to confirm or disconfirm. _____

Emily's Inner Process and Attunement

1. Signals that hint at emotional experience on the leading edge: Emily identifies:
   a. Verbal: pain, injustice, really intense, unanswered questions linger, comes out outbursts of
      rage;
   b. Non-verbal: tone voice intensifies, becoming louder and firmer, as the message intensifies,
      from "not negative," to "very intense," to "very severe," to "I nearly died," to "coming out
      in a rage."
2. Relevant context: Fritz survived a random brutal attack. He has many unanswered questions.
   Emily hears how important it has been for Fritz to minimize his trauma as the best way he knew
   how to manage the intensity, without becoming vengeful.
3. Leading-edge emotion: Emily chooses these words to capture her inference of the leading-edge
   emotion: *Injustice and rage. This was not right! I did not deserve this life-threatening attack!*
   Emily senses a ball of tension and anger gnawing away in her chest as she resonates with
   Fritz's struggle to suppress the incoherence of trauma and intense, unspeakable pain that now
   seems to sneak out in rages.

Emily's Empathic Conjecture
With a tentative tone, Emily links some explicit expressions from the client to a thin slice of experience she hears implied.
   Emily: You struggle to suppress the incoherence of this trauma and your intense, unspeakable
pain sneaks out in rages. I hear that is it so important to you not to be an angry man, and yet, if I
hear you correctly, your clenched fist and trembling jaw are saying, (proxy voice), "This was an
injustice! I nearly lost my life, and it makes no sense how it could have happened! This was not
right! I did not deserve this life-threatening attack!" Do my words match your experience?

Your Strengths and Discoveries about Forming Empathic Conjectures

_____

_____

_____

   More EFIT empathic conjecture workouts are available in the online support material (at rout-
ledge.com/9781032151311).

REFRAMING

Reframing could be considered the backbone of this de-pathologizing, growth-oriented model of therapy. In EFT, the presenting problem is seen to lie, not in one person, but in the rigid, repetitive patterns of interactions in which couples, individuals, and families become caught, in their best attempts to preserve relationships and regulate emotions.

In insecure attachment bonds, people talk and act in code, sending unclear, confusing messages. For example, they push away the person they want close, sometimes inadvertently, with complaints, and sometimes blatantly. Alternatively, people walk away from the person they wish to be close to because closeness feels or has already been dangerous or suffocating.

Reframing provides a validating experience for clients, shifting from a problem mindset to an emotionally-alive, validating attachment frame that brings each client's human goodness and positive relational intentions into the light. As with all EFT micro-skills, reframing is more than a new cognitive mindset offered by the therapist. The intention of a reframing micro-intervention is to *create an experience* of validation, drawing from implicit or explicit attachment intentions and longings that remain hidden in the background by the distressing patterns of interaction.

Reframing is shining an attachment light on the current scene so the longings, vulnerable fears, and good intentions, hidden in the shadows, are seen for what they are. In auditory terms, reframing is highlighting the background musical strains of attachment longings, fears, and intentions, that have been drowned out by the self-protective cacophony of the self-protective cycle of interaction. Framing the repetitive, distressing behaviors or patterns, with attachment, can help clients to move from "helplessness to agency, from negative and dangerous to positive" (Johnson, 2019, p. 70). Attachment reframes can begin to shift views of self and other from critical and hostile to desperate for connection and from cold, aloof, and uncaring to fearful and hurting. This shifts clients from a hopeless, shameful, or accusatory mindset in EFCT to one that acknowledges each partner's goodness and the positive attachment intentions in each of their actions, without ignoring the impact that their unclear and hurtful messages have on their partner.

> ### Salient Questions for EFT Therapists to Ask, When Forming a Reframe
>
> 1. What needs to be reframed? Where could an attachment reframe foster hope or inject new possibilities into an experience of helplessness, or negativity, or pain? Is it an action tendency or a view of self or other that would benefit from a reframe?
> 2. "How do I frame this with an attachment perspective?" That is, how is this dilemma, distress, or problematic interaction, in fact, a dance to hidden strains of attachment themes such as the following: "You are important to me! How can I get your attention?" "How can I protect myself?" "How can I manage alone?"

In EFCT, the reframing micro-skill creates a validating *experience* that a couple's problem is not one partner's deficit, but it is a "between us" dynamic. In EFIT as well, the therapeutic question can be, "How is this a relational response?" How is this internal working model (IWM) relational? Reframing combines with conjecturing to form an important EFT micro-skill known as *catching the bullet,* the topic of the next workout.

The Stage 1 change event of stabilization or de-escalation is essentially *reframing the <u>problem as the pattern</u>* and not one person as the problem. Reactive responses and repetitive patterns are seen to be fueled by core emotions that, when attended to, can become the fuel for change.

Reframes contain an element of conjecture about attachment significance and attachment intentions. Classic EFT reframes for what looks, at first glance, in couple relationships, like negative behaviors of critical pursuit or defensive withdrawal, when held in the light of attachment intentions, are as follows:

- Critical pursuit is reframed as desperate attempts to find the partner and make them respond! Fighting for a response!
- Defensive withdrawal is reframed as being overwhelmed with wanting and failing to get approval, acceptance, and/or appreciation from their partner. Downregulating is also reframed as shrinking away from disapproval or from demands to change who one is.

Insecure attachment strategies can all be framed for their good intentions:

- Anxious hyperactivating can be framed as seeking safety, connection, and responsiveness.
- Deactivating (also known as avoidant suppressing or downregulating) can be framed as survival attempts to move on, without hurting or getting hurt.
- Fearful avoidance, a disorganized strategy, also known as, "Come here; go away," can be framed as seeking support, yet being cautious and judicious of whom to trust.

IWMs or negative labels of self or other can also be reframed in a depathologizing, attachment frame. *Self-attributions* such as "I am inept;" "I'm a failure;" "I'm no good at this" can be seen from an attachment perspective as a core fear of being rejected or of getting hurt or suffocated. They can be reframed as being overwhelmed, or of being frozen in fear of getting it wrong or being pushed aside. *Self-attributions* such as "I'm a maniac;" "I'm a monster;" can be reframed as being frantic to be heard or fighting desperately for a response, all forms of a core fear of abandonment. An *other-attribution* of, "You are crazy," could be reframed as, "When your partner gets so loud, you cannot make sense of what they are saying." An *other-attribution* of, "You are thoughtless and cold," could be reframed as, "When you can't get a response from your partner, their non-response leaves you in the cold, wondering where they are."

How to Formulate Reframes

1. Consider what needs an attachment reframe. Identify where an attachment reframe could foster hope or inject new possibilities into an experience of helplessness or negativity. Is it an action tendency or a view of self or other that needs a reframe?
2. Tune into the attachment threat or attachment longing in the moment. Identify the contextual or attachment threat.
3. EFCT: Find simple words for the hidden attachment story or <u>an attachment reframe</u> of each one's action tendency that becomes the danger cue for the other. (For example, pushing for response, withdrawing or isolating for safety, or from hearing they are causing the other pain.) EFIT: Find simple words for <u>an attachment reframe</u> of the client's action tendency or IWM of self or other. (For example, reframe anxious hyperactivating as genuinely seeking safety and solutions; reframe isolating or avoiding as creatively deactivating for safety.)
4. Formulate a reframe to highlight the hidden attachment messages of mattering to one another that are buried in the distressed interactions. Bring the hopefulness of the attachment story into the light!

EFCT Reframing Workouts

EFCT Reframing Workout 1: Jada and Cornell, Fighting for Response and Retreating from Causing Pain

Context

Jada and Cornell are in a highly escalated pursue-withdraw pattern. She gets what she calls, cruel, mean, and nasty, eventually refusing to talk or touch for days, although she does continue to send angry texts. She is flooded with fears she is not his priority. Cornell rarely fights back but waits for her to let him back again when she is ready.

Client Expressions

JADA: He walks away when I most need him. Every time he walks away it reinforces that he doesn't care. That I am not a priority. Everyone and everything is more important than me. (Cornell smiles, legs start to twitch, and he looks away.) See that smile? He always does this – like he could care less; like I am just a piece of SH…! I mean nothing to him!

CORNELL: She is important to me, but I can't help it really. I smile. I hum. I do all these things when I hear her distress. I get so jittery, like I've lost control of the wheel on a slippery highway. I can't help it – unless I simply walk away.

JADA: All these things, yes – anything but respond to me!!! He's cold and callous. He's so mean.

Your Inner Process and Attunement as You Form a Reframe

1. Identify what needs a reframe. Where could an attachment reframe foster hope or inject new possibilities into an experience of helplessness or negativity? Is it an action tendency or a view of self or other that needs a reframe? _____

_____

2. Tune into the attachment threat or attachment longing for each partner in this moment of reactivity. Identify the threat. _____

_____

3. Find simple words for the hidden attachment story/an attachment reframe of each one's action tendency that becomes the danger cue for the other in EFCT). (For example: pushing for response, withdrawing for safety, or from hearing they are causing the other pain.)

   Jada: _____

   Cornell: _____

Your Reframe

Create a reframe to highlight the hidden attachment messages of mattering to one another that are buried in the distressed interactions and bring the hopefulness of the attachment story into the light:

_____

_____

Emily's Inner Process and Attunement as She Forms a Reframe

1. What to reframe? Emily identifies that an attachment reframe of Jada and Cornell's action tendencies could inject new possibilities into Jada's negative view of self and other and into the pattern in which the couple is caught. Jada takes Cornell's nervous reactions and walking away to mean he is uncaring, cold, and callous; that she is not a priority to him.

2. Attachment threats and longings. Emily identifies that Cornell's smiling and walking away signals an attachment threat to Jada, and she takes it to mean he doesn't care and that he wants to distance himself from her.

   Emily also identifies that Jada's accusations are an attachment threat to Cornell. He responds with self-protective responses of smiling, leg-twitching, and turning away, when in fact Jada is important to him and he hears that he is causing her pain.

3. Simple words for an attachment reframe. Emily identifies the hidden attachment story under the actions that have become the danger cue for the other:

   Jada – is pushing for a response from Cornell.

   Cornell – is agitating and distancing from the overwhelming message that he is hurting Jada, the one he loves.

Emily's Reframe highlights the hidden attachment messages of mattering to one another that are buried in the distressed interactions and brings the hopefulness of the attachment story into the light!

   Emily: Jada, your voice gets louder and louder, not to hurt Cornell, but to get him to hear you and respond; Cornell, her loud voice expressing frustration with you rattles you – you start to shake and smile, not because you don't care or feel cold and nonchalant; you care so much about her distress that you get agitated and finally walk away when you don't know what to do to calm her down; you are overwhelmed to be causing her distress, because she is so important to you, am I getting it? (Pause). And when he walks away to calm his overwhelm that he cannot help you, Jada, you cannot reach him and you don't know he is struggling over your distress and how important you are to him, do you?

Your Strengths and Discoveries

   After reading Emily's responses, compare your responses with hers and see if you discover anything you may want to integrate into your style of creating reframing responses. Also, make a note of your strengths at reframing. The goal here is to shine the attachment light on the darkness and hopelessness to create an experience of hope and agency.

EFCT Reframing Workout 2: Dennis and Hoda, Contextual and Attachment Threats

Dennis, who is white, doesn't understand how unsafe his partner, Hoda feels as a Muslim person of color in their largely white community. They met while he was working abroad and have been together for nearly ten years, but only recently moved to North America. Hoda insists he needs to trust her and believe her that it does not feel safe for her to walk in the community without him. She refuses to walk to the local store without him at her side. Dennis has typically responded with silence, or a slight shrug.

Client Expressions

DENNIS: She's my wife so of course she belongs in this community! How dare people suggest otherwise! I don't want her to feel unsafe, unwelcome here. I want her to know she is always welcome and safe with me and in my country. (Shrugs his shoulders.) We agreed to raise a family here. I need her to feel safe! Sometimes I worry she will never feel at home here!

HODA: The racial slurs, the judgmental glances, he seems to shrug it off. I can't shrug it off. If he cannot understand – then I don't actually feel safe with him either.

Your Inner Process and Attunement

1. Identify what needs an attachment reframe – an action tendency or a view of self or other?

_____

_____

2. Identify and tune into the contextual and attachment threat or longing for each partner.
   For Hoda: _____
   For Dennis: _____
3. Find simple words for the attachment reframe of each one's action tendency that becomes the danger cue for the other.
   Hoda: _____
   Dennis: _____

Your Reframe
Create a reframe that shifts from a hopeless/accusatory mindset to acknowledge each partner's goodness and their positive attachment intentions, without invalidating the real contextual threat:

_____

_____

_____

_____

Emily's Inner Process and Attunement

1. What needs a reframe? Emily identifies that Hoda's lack of safety needs to be framed as a legitimate danger and not a fear that will go away because they want it to. She senses that new possibilities could be injected by reframing Dennis's shrug, and his dismissal of Hoda's fear that increases her lack of safety, as his longing for her to feel safe, and his fear she may never feel safe in his country.

Note: This reframe of his dismissive behaviors as a longing for her to feel safe, will of course not make her feel safer in the community, but it may help to break the escalation between them and help Dennis to see that his longing for Hoda to feel safe (and his underlying fear she may never feel safe) is coming out in ways that make her feel less safe both in the community and in their relationship. The reframe can be part of making it safer for them to openly discuss these contextual dangers, and their attachment fears together.

2. Contextual and attachment threats: Emily senses the following attachment threats or attachment longings for each partner in the face of this contextual danger for Hoda.

    Hoda: alone, misunderstood, and unsafe even with her most important person.

    Dennis: fears Hoda may not ever feel safe in North America and they won't make it as a family together and he could lose her.

    Emily notices that the more Hoda pushes to be believed, the more Dennis dismisses her fear and acts nonchalant and the more unsafe she feels with him and in the community.

3. Simple words for an attachment reframe. Emily identifies these simple words to reframe each one's action tendency:

    Hoda's action tendency is to complain that Dennis doesn't understand; <u>Reframe</u>: Calling Dennis to be her safe person and to believe the reality of the danger she lives.

    Dennis's action tendency is to minimize and dismiss Hoda's fear. <u>Reframe</u>: His best attempt to make it safe for Hoda at this time is to ignore the real danger she experiences. He so desperately wants her to be safe that he misses seeing how dismissing her experience actually increases her sense of danger.

Emily's Reframe

EMILY: It sounds like you both long for the same thing – to feel safe together and to be safe in your community. And Dennis, you find it very difficult to hear that Hoda does experience religious and racial aggression. You miss hearing that your responses make her feel even less safe. Hoda, you get louder and more frustrated, not against Dennis, but to get him to hear you. Dennis, her protests seem to trigger your fear that she will never feel at home here and you dismiss her fears, not because you don't care, but because you are also afraid. Am I getting it? In your circular dance are two people much in love and important to each other, missing hearing your deepest fears, yes?

Your Strengths and Discoveries about Reframing

_____

_____

_____

EFCT Reframing Workout 3: Mindy and Petros, The Threat of Discussing an Attachment Injury

Mindy and Petros are in the de-escalation phase of beginning to repair an attachment injury. They have stabilized and the offending partner, Petros, the withdrawer, has engaged. Three years earlier, Petros admitted he had secretly depleted their savings on a failed business venture. Mindy became frenzied and frantic and Petros withdrew with guilt and fear that Mindy would not want him anymore. So far, they have not been able to have a *healing injuries conversation* to rebuild the trust without triggering their familiar pattern of pursuing/criticizing (Mindy) and withdrawing/minimizing (Petros).

However, since Petros' engagement change event where he asked for assurance that Mindy still wanted him, and received that assurance from Mindy, Petros is willing and confident that he can listen to her pain without backing away. The therapist knows that the path to rebuilding trust includes having engaged dialogues between partners where they can revisit the moment of injury and together create a moment that re-establishes trust. For *a de-escalated partnership to create a re-do* of the moment that shattered the trust between them (Reinna Albornoz, personal communication, October 28, 2023) the nub of the injurious event needs to be named and revisited.

Client Expressions

PETROS: I can listen to your hurt. I am ready to hear from you. I know you were incredibly hurt. We haven't really talked about it. You told me that you care about my well-being, and it means so much to hear that (places his hand on his heart). It gives me hope that we may have a future together where you can forgive me.

The therapist asks Mindy, the injured partner to talk about the shattering moment that broke the trust between them: The moment she "lost her hero" when she found out that Petros had secretly depleted their savings.

MINDY: No, no, I can't believe he could listen. It is too much to remember that time – too much for him to be reminded of all those years of my being an absolute maniac. (Petros, leaning in, looking open to hear from Mindy, looks briefly at the therapist and nods.) It is easier to carry on as though it didn't happen. It's just too much to revisit the maniac I became, (pauses) for years!

Your Inner Process and Attunement

1. Identify what needs a reframe. – action tendency or view of self/other?_____

_____

2. Identify the contextual and attachment threats or attachment longing

    For Mindy: _____

    For Petros: _____

3. Find simple words for an attachment reframe of each one's action tendency that becomes the danger cue for the other.

    Mindy: _____

    Petros: _____

Your Reframe

_____

_____

_____

_____

Emily's Inner Process and Attunement

1. What needs a reframe? Emily identifies that reframing Mindy's view of self as a maniac could inject hope and create more safety.
2. Attachment threats and longings. Emily senses that the therapist's invitation for Mindy to disclose the trust-shattering moment is triggering threat for her. Emily identifies Mindy's fear and shame of recalling how she behaved and hears her fear of hurting Petros if she talks about the event that shattered her trust in him and presumably triggers him to withdraw again. It is threatening to face the shameful memories of her frantic actions (what she calls "being a maniac for years").

   Emily sees Petros' openness to hearing from Mindy. Petros appears not to be triggered in this moment, but rather is genuinely present.
3. Simple words. Emily chooses to reframe Mindy's view of self as a maniac, as being frantic and panicked; in a spin of anger, loss, and fear, not trusting yet that Petros can listen to her pain without withdrawing.

Emily's Reframe

EMILY: Mindy, I hear how badly you feel about how frantic you became for years over Petros' betrayal. Of course, you were panicked, angry, so lost! And I hear how hard it is to believe that Petros is actually leaning in, ready and willing to hear your pain and loss and to learn more about how your rage at him was code for how deeply panicked and hurt you felt.

Your Strengths and Discoveries about Reframing

_____

_____

_____

Another EFCT reframing workout is available in the online support material (at routledge. com/9781032151311).

EFIT Reframing Workouts

If you have come directly to the EFIT workouts in reframing, please read the details about this micro-skill as it is introduced earlier in the EFCT Reframing workouts. The introduction to reframing in the EFCT reframing workouts features reframing as a micro-skill that provides a validating experience for clients, by shifting from a problem mindset to an emotionally-alive, validating attachment frame that brings each client's human goodness and positive relational intentions into the light. As with all EFT micro-skills, reframing is more than a new cognitive perspective offered from the therapist's worldview. It is designed to be a present-moment *experience* of validation and new possibilities, drawing from implicit or explicit attachment intentions and longings that are embedded in the client's story and experience.

EFIT Reframing Workout 1: Luca, Isolating and Withdrawing

Context

Luca, 35, is a gay man who has been crushed by his family since coming out as gay. In particular, his heart is broken from rejection by his twin brother with whom he had always been very close. He struggles with anxiety that he says is disrupting all his relationships, leaving him essentially living an isolated existence. Since many crushing blows from close and extended family members, he has withdrawn from everyone.

Client Expression

Read the client's expression aloud as though you were Luca. Then follow to formulate a depathologizing, attachment reframe.

LUCA: I cannot say what I want to say to people. In fact, I get so anxious I often freeze and I totally lose the words of what I may want to say. It is like a prison of my own making. Sometimes I know I am annoyed but I don't dare feel that. I mute all my feelings, all my thoughts so I don't evoke anyone's wrath or judgement. So I don't risk more judgement on top of the rejection I already feel. There is no way I can take anymore rejection!

Your Inner Process and Attunement as You Form a Reframe

1. Identify what needs a reframe. Where could an attachment reframe foster hope or inject new possibilities? Is it an action tendency or on a view of self or other that needs a reframe?

_____

2. Identify and tune into the contextual or attachment threat or attachment longing: _____

_____

3. Find simple words for an attachment reframe of action tendency or IWMs of self/other. _____

_____

Your Attachment Reframe of Luca's Prison of Isolation

_____

_____

_____

After inserting your reframe, compare your responses with Emily's below. Your inner process and attunement and reframe may be similar to Emily's responses below or they may be very different. Either is ok. The goal here is to practice attuning to see where an attachment reframe could shift a client's experience from helplessness and hopelessness to an emotionally alive experience of hope, agency, positivity and new possibilities.

Emily's Inner Process and Attunement

1. What needs to be reframed? Emily identifies that an attachment reframe of Luca's action tendencies of muting his feelings, silencing his voice, and isolating from others could inject hope into his prison of isolation.
2. Tuning into attachment and contextual threats. Emily identifies Luca's contextual threats of not being accepted in his family for his sexual identity. She also hears the attachment threats of experiencing rejection from important others and fearing more rejection. She identifies his attachment longings for acceptance and safety to engage with others. Those fears and longings are related to his view of others as unsafe and unreliable and to the very real contextual threats as a marginalized person. His view of self is very shaky, feeling unloved, disrespected, and lacking confidence to find the words to speak. His very constricting action tendency it to isolate.
3. Simple words for an attachment reframe. Emily identifies an attachment reframe for his action tendencies of muting his feelings, silencing his voice, and isolating in these simple words: Silencing his voice and isolating are his best and wise attempts at this vulnerable time, to protect himself from more contextual rejection and broken attachment bonds.

Emily's Reframe
To inject some hopefulness into Luca's prison of isolation. Read it out loud to feel the full impact.

EMILY: Your best attempts to protect the relationships with those you love has been to mute your feelings and to silence yourself from saying anything that may put these important relationships in jeopardy, do I get it? It feels safer to live with the rejection you already feel from important people than to risk more rejection if you were to speak up. Costly, and frustrating, but definitely seems to be the wisest path for now, yes? You are choosing what matters most just now – keep yourself safe from more rejection. Something in you says, wisely, "Don't risk openness with these important people. They are not safe."

Your Strengths and Discoveries
After reading Emily's responses, compare your responses with hers and see if you discover anything you may want to integrate into your style of creating reframing responses. Also, make a note of your strengths at reframing. Your reframing may be similar to Emily's or very different – either is ok. The goal here is to shine the attachment light on the darkness and hopelessness to create an experience of hope and agency.

_____

_____

_____

An EFIT seeding attachment workout with Luca is available in online support material (at routledge.com/9781032151311).

EFIT Reframing Workout 2: SuMing, Facing an Impossible Dilemma

Context

SuMing whom you met in a validation workout enters therapy with what she calls "a big struggle in my heart." She feels caught between her heart and her core values. "I hope this struggle doesn't make me a bad person," she ponders. She was married in Hong Kong to her high school sweetheart and has been living in Canada for several years. Her husband has not yet been able to immigrate to Canada, but his arrival is imminent.

Client Expression

SUMING: I know you cannot tell me what to do. My core tells me what is the right thing to do but the external distractions are so powerful – they pull me away. I am very conflicted. I want to be true to my core – to my husband back in Hong Kong, who has not yet been able to immigrate to Canada but I am also in love with a fellow here and conflicted about what to do. Part of my core still loves my husband, but I feel more in love with my new partner. My core tells me three things: I am a good person. Second, I am Chinese – my originality and third (voice breaking) I am my parents' child. I am Chinese means I have to stick with things. And I'm a good person means I need to make the right decision and do the right thing. And I am my parent's child means I need to honor my commitments and not bring shame on the family. I know you cannot tell me what to do. (Pause.) I just hope this struggle doesn't make me a bad person.

Your Inner Process and Attunement

1. Identify an action tendency or a view of self or other to reframe.

_____

_____

2. Identify and tune into the contextual or attachment threat or attachment: _____

_____

3. Simple words for an attachment reframe of her action tendency or view of self/other:

_____

Your Reframe

_____

_____

_____

Emily's Inner Process and Attunement

1. What needs a reframe? Emily identifies that an attachment reframe of SuMing's question of whether her dilemma makes her a bad person (view of self) could inject encouragement into this stuck place.
2. Contextual and attachment threats or longings. Emily attunes to SuMing's sense of an impossible dilemma pulling her in two directions. She identifies both a contextual threat of living in two worlds, with conflicting values; and an attachment threatening experience of being attached to honoring her culture, her parents, and her sense of what being a good person means and also being attached to a man she is not married to.
3. Simple words for an attachment reframe of her action tendency or her models of self/other. Emily identifies: Two good parts, with strong values, and with clear attachment bonds, in conflict; clearly facing the dilemma of being caught between conflicting values and attachments.

Emily's Reframe

EMILY: (Framing SuMing's clarity of her values, her attachments and her emotional dilemma, using SuMing's words, in proxy voice.) These attachments define who you are: I am a good person, I am Chinese, and I am my parents' child. I want to be true to my core and I am in love with a man who is not my husband. What a lot of courage it must take to face this dilemma! You are facing the dilemma head on. You do not yet see a way out, but what touches me is that you are struggling with your dilemma. You are facing very strong emotional pulls in different directions. Either choice, means breaking or stretching some attachment bonds, breaking or stretching some of your values. And now you are continuing to face the dilemma head on without seeing which direction you will go. It is very courageous to be facing this seeming impossible dilemma without losing sense of your conflicting values and attachments.

Your Strengths and Discoveries about Reframing

_____

_____

_____

EFIT Reframing Workout 3: Graham, Caught in a Prison of Hiding Yet Wanting to be Seen

Context

Graham enters therapy in a confusing spin, annoyed with the world. He feels disregarded by everyone who matters to him and describes this as a life-long pattern. He recounts being frequently dismissed by his parents as a young boy, recalling how anxious he felt when he needed to ask for small things like a new toothbrush or a pair of socks. There was a big drama of criticism from his parents and when he cried or looked disappointed about their outbursts, they denied there was any problem. He learned very early to deal with his needs and fears by himself. In fact, he stopped totally asking for anything he needed or wanted and numbed all his anger and indignation. It was safer that way.

Currently, he is in a relationship with a partner who can be verbally aggressive and ignore him for days, while his best friend, demands his help or attention whenever he wants it. He feels suffocated, but incapable of saying no to his friend and hurt and abandoned by his partner. In session, he talks about how he is fed up with not feeling considered by anyone.

Client Expression

GRAHAM: (In an angry tone.) Everyone is just thinking about what they want. My needs don't matter to anyone. They never have! Is it so difficult for anyone to consider what I need or to ask how something impacts me? There is no point in asking for anything! I'm tired of feeling neglected, of feeling invisible. I have this emptiness. (Pauses.) My stomach is completely tight right now. (After looking down in silence for 20 seconds he looks up and begins talking in a calm tone.) I wonder if I'm exaggerating.

Your Inner Process and Attunement

1. Identify what needs an attachment reframe (action tendency or view of self/other?):

_____

2. Identify contextual/attachment threat or longing: _____

_____

3. Simple words for an attachment reframe:

_____

_____

Your Reframe Response

_____

_____

_____

Emily's Inner Process and Attunement

1. What needs a reframe? Emily identifies that the action tendency of shutting down and making himself invisible could benefit from a reframe. His action tendency of questioning if he is exaggerating or minimizing his own experience can also use a reframe.
2. Attachment threats and longings: Emily identifies that Graham's attachment threats of not being seen, not being heard, and not being considered are reinforcing and being reinforced by his action tendencies to hold back and never risk having a voice and making himself seen or assertively asking for his preferences and needs. She also attunes with heaviness to his longings to be seen and responded to in safe ways, in the face of his tendency to discount his own emotions and needs, just as others do to him.

3. Simple words for an attachment reframe. Emily chooses these simple words for an attachment reframe to inject hope and agency: *Staying quiet to be safe, while at the same time wanting to be seen.* Silencing himself and downplaying his own experience are the best ways he knows to survive so far, even as he is beginning to recognize a voice of protest inside of himself.

Emily's Reframe

EMILY: It has always been safer to deal with your longings and needs alone than to feel anger, to protest, and to risk rejection, right? Your body learned to automatically shut down your protests and your anger to protect you, and it just happened now, didn't it? You felt anger, and your stomach tightened, almost as if it said, "Don't go there! it is too dangerous! Don't speak up for yourself!" When others aren't safe you stay quiet, but it is almost like you are looking for a safe way to finally be seen and heard, am I getting it?

Your Strengths and Discoveries about Reframing

_____

_____

_____

Find another EFIT reframing workout in the online support material (at routledge.com/9781032151311).

CATCHING BULLETS TO CONTAIN AGGRESSION

As was mentioned in the introduction to the reframing workouts, reframing combines with conjecturing to form an important EFT micro-skill known as *catching the bullet*. Catching a bullet is an intervention that refers to catching an aggressive, hurtful, or sarcastic remark and deftly reframing it with an attachment conjecture before the stinging impact penetrates the recipient's skin and triggers a self-protective move of distancing or firing back, in EFCT, and in EFIT, before one comment triggers an escalating negative spiral of self-deprecation or imagined attacks from another in the client's mind.

Catching bullets was initially described as an EFCT intervention to protect a partner and prevent a spiral of reactive interactions, when the other partner responded in an aggressive or dismissive manner to their vulnerable disclosure (Johnson, 2004). This intervention, however, can be helpful at any time in therapy when aggressive or dismissive reactivity appears. Catching verbal assaults or harsh disregard with an empathic conjecture reframes hurtful words as genuine disorientation, or fear, or disbelief, and frequently offers a hunch about a hidden positive attachment motive gone awry. This makes it possible to refocus on the process of stabilization or restructuring that got derailed by a harsh reaction.

Whenever they appear, *bullets,* or stinging comments need to be caught or interrupted, and safety needs to be restored. Bullets can appear during any therapist's move with clients or during Stage 1 or 2 of client change. They range from subtle non-verbal messages that could be interpreted in hurtful ways to explicitly harsh comments. There can be *bullets* of aggression and minimization in EFCT from partners and in EFIT from imagined others and between parts of self, all of which require the therapist to interrupt and re-create safety.

The catching bullet workouts are unique in that you are given little time to reflect on your inner process before you jump right in to begin formulating your response. There is an urgent need to catch bullets to stop the pain of aggression or dismissal by interrupting immediately before you know what you will say. Attunement to the attachment threats occurring in the therapy room, courage to step in quickly to interrupt, and hearing your own steady-paced audible reflection of the present process, are the elements that help a therapist to ground themselves to move close to clients in emotionally-dangerous moments with the reprieve of a combined reframe-conjecture, known as catching the bullet.

In the EFCT catching bullet workouts you will practice a micro-skill to block a bitter interruption from jabbing the other partner and triggering a self-protective move of distancing or firing back. In the EFIT catching bullet workouts you will practice interrupting what is frequently a client's automatic self-criticism. By interrupting a client's rapid reactivity, a therapist brings awareness to it and thus has the opportunity to provide an attachment reframe which restores safety, prevents spiraling reactions, and opens the client to possibilities of new action tendencies, new meanings, and new views of self and other.

Inner Process and Attunement for the Catching Bullet Micro-Skill

1. Attune to the attachment threats occurring before you and resonate with the felt sense of the one sending a hurtful message and the one receiving the hurtful message.
2. Immediately act to interrupt the escalation and catch the aggression. Notice your own emotional balance and take a deep breath after interrupting, if not before.

Reframing Aggression with Catching the Bullet Micro-Skill

1. Interrupt escalation.
2. Reflect present process without judgment.
3. Reframe the reactivity by conjecturing at confusion, attachment threat, disorientation, or disbelief.
4. If possible/appropriate: Validate the positive attachment intention.
5. Check with client that the conjecture is accurate.
6. Refocus conversation.

EFCT Catching Bullet Workouts

EFCT Catching Bullet Workout 1: Jake and Rose in Stage 1 Reactivity

Context

Jake and Rose are highly escalated. Ever since Jake described to Rose that while he was at a conference he invited the guest speaker, a woman, to his room for a few drinks, after the bar closed, Rose has been in a frenzied turmoil. Regardless of how many times Jake insists that nothing happened between them, Rose is not comforted. Despite Jake assuring Rose that he told her about it because he felt guilty and because he trusted their relationship and their ability to talk things through that he shared it with her, she cannot be calmed.

Read the clients' expressions below out loud as though you were them. Then follow the prompts to insert your inner process and attunement to formulate a bullet-catching response.

JAKE: I am in despair. I see how much she is hurting. I have made countless changes for her and I don't know what more I can do. I am absolutely desperate!

ROSE: I don't care! I'm too angry to care about your despair! I hear his words, but nothing calms me. I'm not a priority. I am not important. He is careless!

Step in to interrupt and catch the bullet. Follow the prompts to attune to the threat each one is experiencing as the aggressive comments are made and then formulate a bullet-catching intervention.

Your Inner Process and Attunement for the Catching Bullets

1. Attune to the attachment threats occurring before you and resonate with the felt sense of the one sending a hurtful message and the one receiving the hurtful message. _____

_____

2. Immediately act to interrupt the escalation and catch the aggression. Notice your own emotional balance and take a deep breath after interrupting, if not before. _____

_____

Your Catching the Bullet

1. Interrupt escalation: _____

2. Reflect present process without judgment: _____

_____

3. Reframe the reactivity by conjecturing at confusion, attachment threat, disorientation, or disbelief: _____

_____

4. If possible/appropriate: Validate the positive attachment intention. _____

_____

5. Check with client that the conjecture is accurate. _____

6. Refocus conversation. _____

After inserting your responses, compare with Emily's below. They do not need to be the same as hers. They are likely to be different and that is ok.

Emily's Inner Process and Attunement

1. Attachment threats: Emily attunes to the threatening moment of Jake vulnerably describing his despair and his trust they could talk through this together, interrupted by Rose's harsh comment that she doesn't care. Emily also attunes to how Jake's vulnerable statements are an attachment trigger (threat) for Rose. Emily attunes to how both are hurting deeply in the same moment.

2. Interruption and grounding: Emily immediately interrupts, with, "Just a moment please," She takes a breath to ground herself, to release the reactivity she feels, and to attune to each one's sense of threat.

Emily's Bullet-Catching

Read her responses out loud to feel the full impact of her attempt to catch the aggression and to validate two persons under attachment threat.

1. **Interrupt escalation.** She has interrupted.

2. **Reflect present process without judgment.**

   EMILY: Jake you mentioned feeling such despair to see Rose's hurt and not knowing how you can respond to her. And Rose, you stepped in to say you are too angry to care about his despair.

3. **Reframe the reactivity by conjecturing at confusion, attachment threat, disorientation, or disbelief.**

   EMILY: I imagine when your panic and anger are so deep, it feels even worse to hear Jake say he is struggling, when you are struggling so much and long for him to ease your pain, am I getting it?

4. **Validate the positive attachment intention.**

   EMILY: It sounds like in your pain you want Jake to get how much you are hurting, and maybe if he hurts too, he might understand your hurt.

5. **Check with the client for accuracy.**

   EMILY: Am I understanding?

6. **Refocus conversation.**

   EMILY: Can we go back to what you were saying Jake, about how you do see that Rose is still hurting over this event of you inviting the guest speaker to your hotel room for a drink?

Your Strengths and Discoveries

After comparing your response with Emily's, make a note of your strengths to celebrate and/or make a note of what you notice from Emily that you want to integrate into your style.

_____

_____

_____

EFCT Catching Bullet Workout 2: Jorge and Celia, During a Vulnerable Disclosure

Context

Jorge and Celia have stabilized their rather distant withdraw/withdraw pattern. Celia, previously very careful with her every move, has engaged and is sharing quite openly and tenderly with Jorge. In this session, Jorge is deepening his core attachment fears and sharing them with Celia.

Client Expressions

JORGE: So afraid that if I let you see how much I need your reassurance, how much I need you, that you will take one look and say I am not enough of a man. I've tried to share with you but it has never come out right. I was bullied as a kid (pause, lips quivering, face drops.) It's left me feeling so desperately needy for your love; so afraid that if I am not who you want me to be, that I'll lose you, like I did with my ex. She taught me that if I am not exactly who I am supposed to be, that I'm not good enough. I learned I had to be whatever I was supposed to be as a man, or my partner would walk away. Just sharing all this, I'm terrified you'll take one look and shut me out or scoff at me!

CELIA: (Interrupting, with a harsh tone) I'm so mad you've kept it to yourself all these years! You shouldn't give those bullies so much power to still hurt you and frighten you!

Your Inner Process and Attunement for the Catching Bullets

1. Attune to the attachment threats and a felt sense of the one sending a hurtful message and the one receiving the hurtful message. _____

_____

2. Notice your own emotional balance and take a deep breath after interrupting, if not before.

Your Catching the Bullet Response

1. Interrupt escalation: _____

2. Reflect present process without judgment: _____

_____

3. Reframe the reactivity by conjecturing at confusion, attachment threat, disorientation, or disbelief: _____

_____

4. If possible/appropriate: Validate the positive attachment intention. _____

_____

5. Check with client that the conjecture is accurate. _____

6. Refocus conversation. _____

Emily's Inner Process and Attunement

1. Attachment threats. Emily is attuned to how Jorge's disclosure is so new for Celia that she appears threatened he has not shared this before. She is also attuned to Jorge's likely sense of threat that his worst fear is coming true: Celia is not happy with what he just tried to share.
2. Interruption and grounding. "Let's slow down here," Emily introjects. Then she takes a deep breath and attunes to how threatened they must both be in this moment.

Emily's Catching the Bullet Micro-Skill

1. **Interrupt escalation.** Emily has stepped in to stop the conversation.
2. **Reflect present process without judgment.**
   EMILY: Jorge just shared some of his big fears that he has never shared before and you quickly stepped in to say, "Wait a minute, why haven't you told me this a long time ago?"
3. **Reframe the reactivity by conjecturing at confusion, attachment threat, disorientation, or disbelief.**
   EMILY: It seems that it is quite a shock for you to hear him talk so openly about how much he needs you and how afraid he is that if you see how much he needs you, that you may turn away or scoff at him. This is quite a shock for you, like, "Who is this man?" Am I right? (Pause for client to respond.)

No more may be needed but the repetition as follows may be helpful:

   EMILY: He's risking to share a deeper fear than you've ever heard from him. A fear that he could lose you if he shares these fears and needs. So painful to hear that he still hurts, that you step in to stop his pain and you don't know what else to say except to tell him not to let them keep hurting him. You almost miss his greatest fear of *you* shutting him out or scoffing at him. So painful to hear what he has endured, yes? But he is sharing it with you, his most important one, right now, and you are letting him see how hard it is for you to hear what he has endured!
4. **Validate the positive attachment intention.**
   EMILY: I can see that without wanting to push him away it is painful to hear that he has never shared this with you before, yes? And it must also be a little difficult to believe, yes? (Checking that the conjecture is accurate.)
5. **Refocus conversation.**
   EMILY: (After Celia confirms she is in reacting in shock, not to frighten him, but that she is genuinely confused and a bit disoriented.) Can we go back to this new, vulnerable disclosure Jorge was exploring?

Your Strengths and Discoveries about Catching Bullets

_____

_____

_____

EFCT Catching Bullet Workout 3: Catching a Bullet of Racial Aggression with Tricia and Noah

Context

Tricia and Noah are a biracial couple. Tricia is White and her partner, Noah is Black. Tricia is quite unwilling to understand the discrimination that Noah experiences, wishing he could ignore it and that ignoring it would make the contextual threats go away. Many of their arguments appear to intensify the attachment and contextual threats.

Client Expressions

NOAH: She doesn't believe me. I get treated badly even in the grocery store and I refuse to go back to the bar she likes after what happened last time.

TRICIA: I wish he could just man up and be proud of his blackness! Why does he always want to avoid the venues I like to visit? Don't give your power away. It hurts me that you get so upset about these things!

Your Inner Process and Attunement for Catching Bullets

1. Attune to the attachment and cultural threats and resonate with a felt sense of the one sending and the one receiving the hurtful message. _____

_____

2. Notice your own emotional balance and take a deep breath after interrupting, if not before.

Your Catching a Bullet Response

1. Interrupt escalation: _____

2. Reflect present process without judgment: _____

_____

_____

3. Reframe the reactivity by conjecturing at confusion, attachment threat, disorientation, or disbelief: _____

_____

_____

4. If possible/appropriate: Validate the positive attachment intention. _____

_____

5. Check with client that the conjecture is accurate. _____

6. Refocus conversation. _____

Emily's Inner Process and Attunement

1. Attachment and cultural threats: Emily attunes to the threatening moment for Noah that Tricia has not only dismissed his experience; she has attacked it. While she realizes Tricia is also threatened somehow, her denial is further aggression toward Noah and must be stopped.
2. Interruption and grounding: Emily immediately interrupts, with "Just a moment please," and takes a breath to ground herself, to release the reactivity she feels, and to attune to each one's sense of threat.

Emily's Bullet-Catching Process

Read aloud to feel the full impact of her validating two persons under attachment threat.

1. **Interrupt escalation.** Emily: Excuse me, Tricia.
2. **Reflect present process without judgment**.

    EMILY: Noah is describing his real experience of a very hurtful recurring experience – one he's lived time and time again as a black man. It may be so difficult for you to hear, Tricia, that you jump in to stop his story, but I need to stop you and make room for Noah to be heard. (Gives Noah the opportunity to say more.)
3. **Reframe the reactivity by conjecturing at confusion, attachment threat, disorientation, or disbelief.**

    EMILY: When Noah describes the hurtful experiences he lives as a black man, you jump in quickly to say, "Don't get so upset about *these things* – as if they were small matters. I imagine you don't mean to hurt him even more by downplaying his very real, daily experience. Am I getting it? It is very difficult, as a white woman, to begin to understand the adversity your husband copes with every day, so let's slow down, can we? Let's take time to really hear his very important experience. Then we'll come back to hear from you what makes it difficult to listen to his experience without quickly jumping in with your perspective. (Here Emily has checked for understanding, validated her positive intention, and refocused back on Noah's story.)

Your Strengths and Discoveries about Catching Bullets

_____

_____

_____

Find two additional EFCT catching bullet workout in the online support material (at routledge. com/9781032151311)

EFIT Catching Bullet Workouts

As was mentioned in the introduction to catching bullets, bullet catching in EFIT is frequently a deliberate interruption of what is frequently a client's automatic, pattern of self-criticism. By interrupting a client's automatic process, the therapist brings awareness to it and thus has the opportunity to provide an attachment reframe which then opens the client to new possibilities.

The first two examples of catching bullets in EFIT are catching aggression toward self, sometimes very subtle, and sometimes quite blatant. The third example is of imagined aggression from an imaginal other. The need for this micro-skill during encounters with imaginal others will become more clear in Part 2 of the book where you have the opportunity to explore shaping encounters.

EFIT Catching Bullet Workout 1: Martha, Cultural Aggression Against Self

Context

Martha, the single mother of a non-verbal 18-year-old son who lives with autism is facing important post-high-school decisions for him. She is timid and frightened for her son and overwhelmed with the power structures of the school and the social service system. She has little support and feels no one understands her fears and responsibilities. Each time she attempts to speak with the school personnel and social service supports, she feels dismissed and devalued. She is beginning to feel no one really cares what happens to her son or to her, for that matter.

Client Expression

MARTHA: We have such important decisions to make, and I don't know what will be best for him! I'm convinced most parents of children on the spectrum handle the parental shame so much better than I do. So many parents seem to carry themselves with such dignity as advocates for their child, while I mouse away in shame and feel I don't belong. And when I try, I get brushed off or demeaned.

Your Inner Process and Attunement

1. Attune to the attachment threats and a felt sense of her present-moment experience. _____

_____

2. Notice your own emotional balance and take a deep breath after interrupting, if not before.

_____

Step in to Stop the Aggression Against Self. Your Catching the Bullet

1. Interrupt escalation: _____

2. Reflect present process without judgment: _____

_____

3. Reframe the reactivity by conjecturing at confusion, attachment threat, disorientation, or disbelief: _____

_____

4. If possible/appropriate: Validate the positive attachment intention. _____

_____

5. Check with client that the conjecture is accurate. _____

6. Refocus conversation. _____

Emily's Inner Process and Attunement

1. Attachment threats: Emily attunes to the contextual threat of marginalization that Martha experiences as a parent of a neurodiverse son. She attunes to Martha feeling daunted and dwarfed by the system and feeling she doesn't belong. She hears it is difficult to trust that she is seen or heard or that her voice is wanted.
2. Interruption and grounding: Emily softly interrupts, with, "Just a moment please," and takes a breath to ground herself and attune to Martha's sense of threat.

Emily's Bullet-Catching Process

1. **Interrupt escalation.** Emily: Martha, can we slow down?
2. **Reflect present process without judgment**.
   EMILY: You have just described facing big decisions for your son and how difficult it is to get the school and social service systems to respond to you and then you dropped into comparing yourself with other parents and falling short.
3. **Reframe the reactivity by conjecturing at confusion, attachment threat, disorientation, or disbelief.**
   EMILY: When you are facing such challenging decisions for your son without the support you may need, it is so easy to slip into questioning your style or even your own worth, am I getting how it goes?
4. **Validate the positive attachment intention.**
   EMILY: I hear how overwhelming these decisions can be and when it is difficult to reach out for others' support or there seems to be no one to reach for, it is easy to overlook the power and the dignity of your love as a mom.
5. **Check with the client for accuracy.**
   EMILY: Am I understanding?
6. **Refocus conversation.**
   EMILY: Can we go back to exploring the barriers and the fears you experience when it comes to advocating for him?

Your Strengths and Discoveries

After comparing your response with Emily's, make a note of your strengths to celebrate and/or make a note of what you notice from Emily that you want to integrate into your style.

_____

_____

EFIT Catching a Bullet Workout 2: Yousef, Contextual and Self Aggression

Yousef suffered a racially motivated attack 15 years earlier in a shopping mall. He was out looking for a birthday gift for his one-year-old son. Now his son is turning 16 and Yousef finds he is continually losing his patience with him. He feels that his angry outbursts don't fit the situation but are somehow related to his unprocessed trauma from the attack over a decade ago.

Client Expression

YOUSEF: I have disregarded my hate, my pain, the helplessness of the guy on the ground being beaten. I have ignored the injustice against me. I feel good that I was able to do this and didn't become a vengeful, social beast. I'm proud of that but at the same time, I feel that this was not the right way. I didn't want to get revenge, so I internalized my pain and my hatred in a way that hurt me a lot. It still hurts! That wasn't right. I did not handle this right! And now I'm having all these random outbursts.

Your Inner Process and Attunement for Catching Bullets

1. Attune to the attachment threats and felt sense of his present-moment experience: _____
_____

2. Notice your own emotional balance and take a deep breath after interrupting, if not before. __
_____

Your Catching the Bullet. Although this is not harsh aggression toward himself, how can you catch this bullet of "I didn't do it right"?

1. Interrupt escalation: _____

2. Reflect present process without judgment: _____
_____

3. Reframe the reactivity by conjecturing at confusion, attachment threat, disorientation, or disbelief: _____
_____

4. If possible/appropriate, validate the positive attachment intention. _____
_____

5. Check with client that the conjecture is accurate. _____

6. Refocus conversation. _____

Emily's Inner Process and Attunement

1. Attachment threats: Emily attunes to the contextually threatening moment of being attacked, unsafe, and physically harmed, likely because he is ethnically from a non-dominant group. She also attunes to what seems to be a more active threat for Yousef in the present moment; that is, he is troubled by his "random outbursts" in the present and slightly judging himself for how he handled this trauma, by ignoring his pain and hatred.

2. Interruption and grounding: Emily immediately interrupts, with "Just a moment please" and takes a breath to ground herself and release the reactivity she feels that he was mercilessly attacked and needs to carry all this unprocessed emotion which continues to threaten him. She

wants to focus on the present dilemma for Yosef today and to interrupt his automatic reaction to begin to judge himself for not handling his hatred and pain in the right way 15 years ago.

Emily's Bullet-Catching Process

1. **Interrupt escalation**. Emily: Yousef,…
2. **Reflect present process without judgment.**
    EMILY: You talk about feeling proud that you have disregarded your anger and not become a vengeful person and then you add, "But this was not right." You are quick to say that you did not handle this in the right way.
3. **Reframe the reactivity by conjecturing at confusion, attachment threat, disorientation, or disbelief.**
    EMILY: I hear what sounds almost like confusion. You lived all these years, true to your values of not becoming vengeful, and yet today you are noticing that you are still hurting and sensing that perhaps there is a different way to listen to your hurt. You sense there could be another way to respond to this horrific event you survived, yes?
4. **Validate the positive attachment intention.**
    EMILY: It sounds almost like you want to find a safe way to openly face the injustice you experienced and to safely respond to it.
5. **Check with the client for accuracy.**
    EMILY: Am I understanding?
6. **Refocus conversation.**
    EMILY: Can we go back to what you were saying about the injustice that you endured?

Your Strengths and Discoveries about Catching Bullets

_____

_____

_____

EFIT Catching Bullet Workout 3: Simona, Receiving a Bullet from an Imagined Other

Context

Simona, in a Stage 2 change event is deeply engaged in revisiting the lasting impacts of her childhood trauma. Her pervasive sense of her mother is that of a harsh, punitive woman who minimizes and denies her experience. She recalls a very humiliating incident where her mother laughed at her and teased her in front of the extended family, but she knows her real mother will deny that ever happened.

Client Expression

SIMONA: I cannot see my own goodness. I can just see my mother wagging her finger at me with that sickly sweet smile, in a very aggressive tone saying, "You are making too much of this, Simona Rose! I did not treat you as badly as you remember. I certainly never made fun of you in front of your grandparents and the extended family!"

Your Inner Process and Attunement

1. Attune to the attachment threats and resonate with a felt sense of her present-moment experience: _____

2. Notice your own emotional balance and take a deep breath after interrupting, if not before. __

_____

Your Catching the Bullet

1. Interrupt escalation: _____

2. Reflect present process without judgment: _____

_____

3. Reframe the reactivity by conjecturing at confusion, attachment threat, disorientation, or disbelief: _____

_____

4. If possible/appropriate: Validate the positive attachment intention. _____

_____

5. Check with client that the conjecture is accurate. _____

6. Refocus conversation. _____

Emily's Inner Process and Attunement

1. Attachment threats: Emily attunes to the threatening, unsafe moment of being laughed at in front of the extended family and the even more threatening sense presently, that her mother who injured her denies that it happened and thus blocks the potential repair of the injurious event.

2. Interruption and grounding: Emily immediately interrupts, with "Ouch! Let's slow down here, please," and takes a breath to ground herself, to release the reactivity she feels toward Simona's mother, and to attune to Simona's sense of threat from a very present, imaginal, harsh mother who blocks her from seeing her own goodness.

Emily's Bullet-Catching Process

1. **Interrupt escalation.**
   EMILY: Ouch! Let's slow down here, please.
2. **Reflect present process without judgment.**
   EMILY: You began to recall with such clarity, this humiliating, painful incident and then suddenly you hear your mother's harsh voice interrupting you and you see her accusatory finger denying your experience.
3. **Reframe the reactivity by conjecturing at confusion, attachment threat, disorientation, or disbelief.**
   EMILY: This must be very confusing. Must be difficult to feel confident in your memories or at least very, very frustrating that, even in your imagination, your mother does not let you tell the story without interruption, yes?

4. **Validate the positive attachment intention.**

   EMILY: You deserve to describe the pain you endured and are feeling to this day, and it is difficult to stay focused on your experience, when your imaginal mother interrupts, yes? I sense a longing to trust that your memories are valid and if at all possible, to experience that your mother, if not in real life, at least in your imagination, could listen and hear what you have to say. If she could listen, that would help to validate your goodness, just may be, yes?

5. **Check with the client for accuracy.**

   EMILY: Am I understanding?

6. **Refocus conversation.**

   EMILY: Can we go back to how this punitive sense of your mother is impacting your sense of self today? How difficult it is to see your own goodness?

Your Strengths and Discoveries about Catching Bullets from an Imagined Other

_____

_____

_____

Bullets from Therapists: Missteps or Micro-Aggressions

When a therapist realizes they have committed or may have inadvertently committed a microaggression, an adaptation of the EFT micro-skill of catching the bullet can be helpful. It doesn't erase the zinger a client may have already experienced, but it is the kindest move a therapist can make after a misstep. Interrupt yourself; acknowledge what you just did; ground yourself, with a breath to release the reactivity you may feel toward yourself and refocus on the client. Attune and evoke how the client is doing, so your acknowledgement and your apology do not turn the focus on you.

Examples of faux pas or microaggressions from the therapist follow, together with a therapist's best attempt to catch the aggression or message of exclusion and restore safety for the client. There is space for you to insert your preferred way of catching the bullet if you make a similar faux pas. Your style may fit much better for you. What is important as in all workouts in this book, is that you are attuned to your client and your own inner process in the moment and are prepared for how to respond with the most respect, empathy, and personal responsibility in these unfortunate moments. Our own bullets remind us that we cannot be perfect. We can simply be present and carry the weight of our own responsibility without burdening the client in any way to make us feel better.

Therapist Misstep Workout 1

A therapist realizes they just implied to a client that they don't belong here, by asking, "Where are you from?"

Your Version of Catching the Bullet to Repair the Rupture. _____

_____

_____

Emily's Version of Catching the Bullet to Repair the Rupture.

EMILY: (Pauses immediately.) I am sorry. It was wrong of me to ask where you are from. No excuse. I am glad we are here together today. Please feel free to let me know anything that will make it safe and comfortable for you here and feel free to give me any feedback you have if my words are hurtful. I am eager to get to know you. How are you doing now?

Therapist Misstep Workout 2

A therapist makes an assumption, upon seeing a woman's wedding ring, that she is married to a man and asks, "Did you invite your husband to come with you to therapy?" immediately the therapist realizes that may have been a microaggression.

Your Version of Catching the Bullet to Repair the Rupture. _____

_____

_____

Emily's Version of Catching the Bullet to Repair the Rupture.

EMILY: (She pauses immediately.) I'm sorry, I should have asked, "Did you ask your partner to join you in therapy?" What would you like to tell me about your experience or your hopes?

After any such faux pas that could convey aggression or exclusion, you can acknowledge a mistake but do not wait for a client to tell you it is ok or to "accept your apology." When we hurt someone inadvertently, we hold the pain of that moment and then we move on to communicate respect and empathy and to foster and monitor the safety of the therapeutic alliance. Another therapist misstep workout is available in the online support material (at routledge.com/9781032151311).

SEEDING ATTACHMENT

Seeding attachment is a type of conjecture – an inference that simultaneously heightens and validates a client's core fear, while at the same time, seeds an imaginal interpersonal scenario of the soothing antidote to that fear.

   This micro-intervention was originally used during Stage 2 restructuring change events (Johnson, 2004) and began with heightening repetitions of the reach that feels far too difficult and frightening for a partner to make. For example, "You could never, never ever …," followed by an explicit expression of the attachment longing and a description of an antidote comforting interaction.

How to Formulate Seeding Attachment in EFCT

With *seeding attachment*, a therapist describes a scenario of risking, reaching, and receiving comfort – a process that has, up until now, been blocked by fears of rejection or abandonment. For example, "You could never, never ever reach to your partner and say, 'I am afraid that I am too much for you to love', and imagine them responding to you with the love, comfort, and assurance that you crave. You could never, ever imagine receiving that tender response to your fear?" The intervention *seeds,* in the imagination, a picture of secure reaching and responding while also heightening the fear. With this intervention, a vision of the seismic shifts of Stage 2 change is foreshadowed.

Seeding attachment can also be used in Stage 1, particularly in setting goals and envisioning hopes for change, when the change feels very far away. The risk of taking a new step of change is not heightened as in Stage 2, but the seed of imagining an antidote comforting response to clients' core longings, distress, and/or fears is planted. The manifestation of attachment goals and longings, which contain new views of self as lovable, worthy, and competent, and of others as accessible, responsive, and reliable, can be imagined in specific and emotionally alive scenarios.

EFCT Seeding Attachment Workouts

The first two EFCT seeding attachment workouts are Stage 2 examples; the final workout is a Stage 1 example.

EFCT Seeding Attachment Workout 1: Cass and Bryson Toward Withdrawer Engagement

Context

Cass and Bryson have an ongoing argument. Bryson pursues with demands and Cass withdraws. Bryson insists that it is not Cass he is upset with when he walks into a room that is not in perfect order and cleanliness. It is his sense that if he really mattered to Cass, she would care about the neatness and tidiness that are so important to him. They have de-escalated and the therapist is helping Cass engage more deeply in expressing her core fears, toward stepping more assertively into the relationship.

Client Expression

CASS: It's one of those looks that really throw me. When he walks into a room and his eyes widen and his brow furrows, I see judgement and I feel through and through that he's upset with me. He tells me it's not about me. But my heart starts to pound and my stomach starts to churn. I already know in my head that he believes that that look is not against me (laughs) but I see one of those looks and I'm gone – out of the way – feeling bad and wrong! It's like a fire hose blasts me away!

Follow the prompts to attune to Cass' fear in this de-escalated couple. This will help you to create a *seeding attachment* intervention that brings to life the possibility of Cass risking to move out of her withdrawal position toward Bryson and receiving the antidote response from him that will calm her fear.

Your Inner Process and Attunement

Identify Cass' core fear or implied longing and attachment need:

Resonate in your body to how you imagine that fear or unmet longing must feel:

_____

Find words to describe an interpersonal antidote to her core fear; how she could reach and the partner could respond in a way that would transform that fear:

_____

_____

Your Seeding Attachment Intervention

Find the words to form a seeding attachment intervention, by validating the fear and with repetition, heightening both the fear and the antidote to the fear. Link an expression of the fear to a picture of receiving the very response that would soothe that fear. As with all conjectures, be tentative, to check with the client that this is fitting for them: You may begin with, "You could never imagine;" or "You could never, ever…." _____

_____

_____

Emily's Inner Process and Attunement

Core fear/longing: Emily identifies Cass' core fear as feeling sheer rejection, feeling blasted away from Bryson by one look of disapproval. She identifies that Cass longs for Bryson's acceptance of her as she is.

Bodily resonance: As Emily resonates in her own body to how she imagines that would feel, she has a sense of cold tingles running through her entire body to see a look which to Cass has come to mean she is somehow bad, and wrong in Bryson's eyes, and is feeling pushed away with disgust.

Interpersonal antidote: Emily identifies that the perfect antidote to this repetitive stuck point would be if Cass could step toward Bryson and tell him about her fear and he would respond with assurance at the moment that she risks disclosing her fear.

Emily's Seeding Attachment

Read it out loud to feel the full impact of the heightened fear and the heightened vision of how, specifically, the relevant other can soothe or transform this fear.

EMILY: You would never go to Bryson and say, "It's happening! I'm getting that panicky, anxious feeling – afraid you don't understand me. Afraid you don't really care. The countertops are not spotless and all I see is a big sign on your face that says that I don't matter to you."
You can't ever imagine sharing that? (voice is tentative) That feels too small, too petty, yes? So, he never gets to hear about your anxious stomach, your pounding heart, does he? (Wait for client confirmation.) So very frightening to see that look on his face and immediately be filled with the fear, "I'll never be enough for him. Never, ever can I be the sort of partner he needs." You could never, ever imagine when this fear is blasting you way, way across the room that you could go to him and ask him to assure you it is you he wants? You could never imagine him responding with assurance if you asked? Do I understand?

Your Strengths and Discoveries

Compare your inner process and response with Emily's. Your response may be very different from hers and that is ok. The important thing is to experiment with being aware of your inner process and attunement and with attempting to seed an imagined shift toward attachment security. After comparing your response with Emily's, make a note of your strengths to celebrate and/or make a note of what you notice from Emily that you want to integrate into your style.

EFCT Seeding Attachment Workout 2: Jill and Zev Toward a Softening

Context

Jill and Zev have de-escalated a very well-entrenched, protective pattern of Jill protesting with increasing frantic calls for Zev to be more engaged in the relationship and Zev freezing, shaking, and going cold, met with occasional backlashes of anger and then more disappearance.

In the engagement change event, Zev showed up with assertive and vulnerable clarity. Having always struggled to ask for anything for himself, he reached a place he where could say to Jill:

> I do need your acceptance I need to know I am good enough for you; that I am not a disappointment to you! My despair is caused by my feelings of inadequacy which comes directly from things you say. My radar is always on. Always on guard for signs that you are displeased with me.

He wept, he shook, he hesitated, and finally in an assertive, clear voice, said, "I need your help to let me know I am o.k. You're o.k., we're o.k. I need you to help me deal with this fear."

Jill, still reeling with shock, exclaims, "I thought it was all anger! I didn't know you were afraid of anything – especially not afraid of disappointing me! I just thought you were distant, angry and I couldn't reach you." Now that Jill understands that Zev was not distancing out of anger and nonchalance but out of fear of disappointing her, she feels calmer, more compassionate, and more assured of his presence.

Jill is increasingly experiencing a new view of other. Zev remains present and engaged, however, her fears of view of self, as needing far too much, are spiking! As Jill expands and deepens her core fears she is terrified at the enormity of her need for Zev's assurance and deeply ashamed for having ranted at him so relentlessly for years. She begins her softening as follows:

Client Expression

JILL: Zev seems so different now – more caring, more present. All I have ever wanted is to feel that you see me and hear me and are with me. I have that now, but I still have a huge fear that I need you too much. I've always felt I was being punished for needing too much. And I'm so ashamed – needing you so much – yet all the lashing out I've done! It's pathetic really. How can you possibly want me? I get a sheer panic that I don't feel I deserve your company when I am so desperate! Too humiliated to ask – embarrassed – never showed this to anyone before.

Your Inner Process and Attunement

Identify Jill's core fear or implied longing and attachment need:

_____

Resonate in your body to how you imagine that fear or unmet longing must feel:

_____

Find words to describe an interpersonal antidote to her core fear; how she could reach and the partner could respond in a way that would transform that fear:

_____

_____

_____

Your Seeding Attachment Intervention

Find the words to form a seeding attachment micro-skill, by validating the fear and with repetition, heighten both the fear and the interpersonal antidote to the fear. Link an expression of the fear to a picture of receiving the very response that would soothe that fear. Be tentative and check with Jill whether your words are fitting for her: You may begin with, "You could never imagine;" or "You could never." _____

_____

_____

Emily's Inner Process and Attunement

Core fear/longing: Emily identifies Jill's core fear as one of being undeserving of Zev's love; feeling humiliated at how much she needs him, ashamed for how harshly she has treated him all these years, out of desperation, and fearful she is too much to be loved.

Resonance: As Emily resonates in her own body with how this must feel for Jill, she feels herself shrinking and curling up inside. She also senses a burning sensation in her cheeks for how difficult it is for Jill to recall her harsh and frenzied attempts to get Zev to engage.

Interpersonal antidote: Emily is confident that if Jill can take the ultimate risk of reaching out to Zev who clearly values and loves her to ask for his assurance that he will respond with tenderness. She knows the impact of Zev's response will be heightened exponentially if Jill can take the risk of asking for it.

Emily's Seeding Attachment Intervention

EMILY: (With a tentative tone) You can't imagine – could never, ever imagine that Zev would take one look at this beautiful vulnerable Jill and want to come in and assure you how much he loves you. You can't imagine he loves this desperate Jill who gets so panicked and feels so alone; who so desperately needs him and his comfort. You could never, ever show this vulnerable, needy self to Zev and ask him if he can love you like this. Can't imagine that he would love this part of you and want to reach in and comfort you, and assure you how previous you are to him! Is that right?

Your Strengths and Discoveries about Seeding Attachment

_____

_____

_____

EFCT Seeding Attachment Workout 3: Goal Setting with Mara and Annette

Context

Mara and Annette are a white, lesbian couple in early EFT therapy. Mara self-identifies on the Autism spectrum. She faults herself for not being a good communicator and not knowing how to multitask and or to show Annette that she is number one, despite her preoccupation with managing a business. She automatically withdraws under stress, sometimes followed by outbursts of anger. She prides herself on being self-sufficient, having lived without parental care since she was 14.

Annette is an anxious pursuer who also withdraws to give Mara space and to protect herself from the outbursts Mara tends to have when she is overloaded with work. "I slink away to give Mara space when I see her getting agitated," says Annette. When Mara gets frustrated or angry, Annette is flooded with flashbacks of the physical and sexual abuse she survived as a child.

Recently, Mara has been exceptionally present to care for Annette since Annette suffered a workplace injury. As Anette is recovering, she fears that Mara will disappear again after she no longer needs physical care. Mara insists she does not want to disappear and does not want Annette to be afraid of her frustration. "But I get overloaded and I do need her help. It is complicated. I never want to frighten her with my anger."

In this early session, the therapist invites each partner to identify their hopes and goals for therapy.

Client Expression

ANNETTE: I want to talk about our lack of intimacy and closeness in general. We work together. She owns a business. My biggest hope out of therapy is that when I am able to return to work, she won't take her frustration out on me anymore and then withdraw in anger. And that we can get our sex life back.

Follow the prompts to attune to Annette's core longing. The prompts will help you to form a *seeding attachment* intervention that can help in the goal-setting process. This is early EFT therapy, so you can use this as an opportunity to paint a picture of the attachment longing you hear in the goals Annette has described, worded in a way that may also fit for Mara.

Your Inner Process and Attunement

Identify Annette's core attachment longing and/or fear:

_____

Your bodily resonance of how that fear or unmet longing must feel:

_____

Find words to describe an interpersonal antidote to her core fear:

_____

_____

_____

Your Seeding Attachment Intervention

_____

_____

_____

Emily's Inner Process and Attunement

Core fear/longing: Emily identifies Annette's core fear of Mara's angry outbursts and her withdrawal. She identifies her core longing to feel safe with Mara and to have more emotional and sexual intimacy.

Resonance: As Emily attunes to Annette's core fears of Mara's anger and her withdrawal and to her longings for safety and intimacy, she resonates with a hollow, emptiness in her own core – longing to feel safe and close and wanted by her partner, yet fearing distance and push-away anger.

Interpersonal antidote: Emily hears an implied longing to be safe together though they describe the picture of safety differently just now. She finds these words to seed a picture of safety, envisioning a goal to work toward: Mara feels wanted and safe to ask for support and Annette knows how to support Mara so she is not so stressed and caught up in her own world but is comfortable being close to Annette.

Emily's Seeding Attachment Intervention

Emily: (In a tentative tone of voice, checking if this picture of safety that she hears implied in their longings, fits for each one of them.) It sounds like you both long to feel safe and comfortable together – where Mara, you can comfortably come to Annette for support in your frustrating moments and where Annette you feel safely needed and wanted and appreciated by Mara. I hear that your picture of this kind of safety, Annette, also includes feeling warm and turned on and sexy with each other, though I know these are not Mara's words at this time. Am I hearing accurately the hopes and longings you each have?

Your Strengths and Discoveries about Seeding Attachment

_____

_____

_____

An additional EFCT seeding attachment workout, imagining attachment injury repair, is available in the online support material (at routledge.com/9781032151311).

EFIT Seeding Attachment Workouts

Although this micro-skill was designed for EFCT, it is also very useful in EFIT. *Seeding attachment* is a type of conjecture that can be used in EFIT to simultaneously heighten and validate a client's core fear, longing, or unmet need, while at the same time planting a seed of an imaginal interpersonal scenario of a soothing antidote to that fear. If you have come directly to the EFIT workouts, you may want to read the introduction to *seeding attachment* preceding the EFCT seeding attachment workouts. Similar to EFCT, with the *seeding attachment* micro-skill in EFIT, a therapist describes a scenario of the client's heightened core fear or longing, fully alive and expressed, being met with and transformed by an interpersonal response.

How to Form Seeding Attachment in EFIT

- Identify the client's core fear and implied longing/attachment need.
- Resonate in your body to your felt sense of the client's core emotion.
- Find words for core fear or longing and an interpersonal antidote response from a significant other who could be the therapist, an imaginal other, or the interpersonal reach and response could be between parts of self.
- Heighten and combine the fear, longing, or unmet need with the antidote interpersonal response. The two together (heightened core emotion and soothing response) become a powerful *seed of attachment* that plants hope.

The EFIT Seeding attachment workouts contain one in Stage 1 with seeding attachment security as part of goal setting, and two in Stage 2 sessions where seeding attachment is used, first as part of an engagement change event and secondly as a softening change event. Find another Stage 1 EFIT seeding attachment workout in the support material online (at routledge. com/9781032151311).

EFIT Seeding Attachment Workout 1: Shaping a Goal with Sahra, Swinging Between Hyperactivating and Numbness

Context

Initially, Sahra says she is getting weary of the highs of anxiety and the lethargy of depression. She is caught in a fearful avoidant pattern, annoyed with herself for flipping between agitation, anxiety, and flat numbness. Her hopes for therapy are to stabilize the highs and lows, to stop the flashbacks of her ex's violence, to heal her broken heart from the harsh men she has had in her life, to stop feeling so anxious, and to somehow get a grip on her untouchable grief over her mother's death far off in Ukraine when Sahra she could not be with her.

Client Expression

SAHRA: What's the point in noticing my pain? I'm afraid it will hurt even more if I feel it or share it. I'm afraid no one cares to listen anyway! I feel I let my guard down a little too much. I trusted a few people I should never have trusted. Now I see

I shouldn't have even trusted me! Better to put those stories back in storage and grow a thicker skin again. Toughen up like I learned to do a long time ago! Maybe it is better not to feel? But I do feel and I need to sort out all this pain or it will destroy me.

Follow the prompts to attune to Sahra's core longing. The prompts will help you to prepare to create a *seeding attachment* intervention that can help in the goal-setting process. This is early EFT therapy, so you can use this as an opportunity to paint a picture of the attachment longing you hear in what Sahra has shared.

Your Inner Process and Attunement

Core fear/longing: Identify the client's core fear or implied longing and attachment need:

_____

Resonance: Resonate in your body to how you imagine that fear or unmet longing must feel:

_____

Interpersonal antidote: Find words to describe an interpersonal antidote to the core fear or longing. The interpersonal response could be from the therapist, an imaginal other, or the interpersonal reach and response could be between parts of self.

_____

_____

_____

Your Seeding Attachment Intervention

Find the words to form a seeding attachment intervention that will help with goal setting. Combine heightening both the fear and the antidote to the fear. Link an expression of the fear to a picture of receiving the very response that would soothe that fear. As with all conjectures, be tentative and check with the client whether your words are fitting for them: You may begin with, "You long for..."

_____

_____

_____

Emily's Inner Process and Attunement

Core fear/longing: Emily identifies the core fear as total aloneness/abandonment and fear of noticing and feeling the losses and grief she feels. There is an implied longing for safety and for sorting out her pain. It seems there is no safety anywhere just now – neither internal safety to trust herself to make good relationship choices, nor interpersonal safety for support.

Resonance: As Emily resonates in her own body to how she imagines that fear of nothing being safe, the experience of abandonment, and a longing for safety must feel for Sahra, her heart is heavy and she feels her entire body tingly, as though she were out in the cold with no protection.

Interpersonal antidote: Emily hears an implied longing to be safe internally; for Sahra to trust her own emotions and decisions and ultimately to be safe with at least some others in her world.

Emily's Seeding Attachment Intervention

EMILY: (In a tentative tone of voice, checking if this picture of longed-for safety that she hears in Sahra's story fits for her.) It sounds like you long to feel safe within yourself and with all the losses and grief you carry. You can't imagine yet, feeling safe to share your pain and to tell your stories out loud. You can't imagine safely sharing your losses and having someone – me for starters – listen and be with you in that pain so you are not alone. It is such a big step to imagine feeling safe enough to share these stories bit by bit as you are ready, until you reach the place where you have some internal and interpersonal safety and trust again.

Your Strengths and Discoveries

Compare your inner process and response with Emily's. Your response may be very different from hers. The important things are to experiment with being aware of your inner process and with attempting to form a seeding attachment micro-skill that combines the core fear with an imagined interpersonal interaction that soothes or transforms that fear – creating an imagined shift toward security. Make a note of your strengths to celebrate and/or what you notice from Emily that you want to integrate into your style. _____

_____

_____

_____

EFIT Seeding Attachment Workout 2: Max's Engagement with an Imaginal Léo

Max has kept emotionally distant from his friend Léo who died in the street-racing crash when they were teenagers. He wants to face his image of Léo, yet he continues to push all the thoughts and memories and feeling of guilt into what he has come to call his *emotional storage boxes*. Several Stage 1 corrective emotional experiences have made it safer for him to own his patterns of minimizing and denying, to cope with his feelings of guilt for denying being the driver of the car that crashed and killed his friend and for surviving when his friend died. He is stabilizing his patterns of avoidance yet remains very hesitant to face an imaginal Léo because that means facing himself as a harmful, guilty person.

Client Expression

MAX: I have to face how badly injured he must have been. I suffered so much damage, but I survived. What his body suffered must have been so much worse. I have to face that I am the one who crashed the car. For so many years, I insisted to myself that I was not the driver!

Your Inner Process and Attunement
Core fear/longing: _____

Your bodily resonance: _____

Interpersonal antidote: Find words to describe an interpersonal antidote, from the therapist, an imaginal other, or an interpersonal reach and response between parts of self. _____

_____

_____

_____

Your Seeding Attachment

_____

_____

_____

Emily's Inner Process and Attunement
Core fear/longing: Emily identifies Max's core fear as terror at fully facing and feeling what happened – specifically how badly his friend was damaged while he was driving a car in a street race.

Resonance: Emily finds that she feels quite numb with a twinge of tension across her chest as she seeks to resonate in her own body with Max. This tension in her chest grows as she imagines Max's terror of facing what happened and longing to survive fully facing the damage to Léo's body and his part in the tragedy that took his friend's life.

Interpersonal antidote: As Emily tries to imagine what interpersonal interaction could be an attachment antidote to Max's terror and guilt, she imagines Max feeling safe to picture an imaginal Léo and perhaps to have an imaginal dialogue with him. Feeling safe to be in his imaginal presence without feeling judgment.

Emily's Seeding Attachment
Emily: You can't imagine picturing Léo and feeling safe to tell him how sorry and responsible you feel for his death. You can't imagine sharing with Léo that you tried to convince yourself and everyone else that you were not the driver, because it was just too hard to face otherwise. You

can't imagine that if you shared how hard this has been on you, that Léo would care about you, is that it? Can't imagine that your good friend would care to hear you tell him how sorry you are that he died that day and how guilty you've felt all the years that you survived. So difficult to picture telling Léo that it's been hard on both of you and that you'd like him to hear from you. So hard to imagine that he could listen to your pain and remorse, and say, "I get it! You're right. We have both struggled here – alone." Very hard to picture that kind of response from Léo, yes?

Your Strengths and Discoveries about Seeding Attachment

_____

_____

_____

EFIT Seeding Attachment Workout 3: Sahra, Preparing for a Softening

Context

Sahra, from Workout 2 above, has stabilized patterns of swinging between hyperactive anxiety and numbing lethargy. She is managing very well without significant attachment support in her life at this time and drawing on friendships where she can. She is having professional successes; however, she continues to carry the weight of "the strong Black woman" stereotype and she admits to feeling exhausted, weak, physically unwell, and experiencing she is of value to others only when she can produce work. The continued social pressure to be strong and productive, combined with ongoing racial discriminatory treatment from some of her colleagues, especially when she is feeling unwell, continue to reinforce the message that as a person of color, she needs to work twice as hard to be seen as half as good.

Client Expression

SAHRA: Where is my value, I wonder some days! It's hard to believe I am of value when I am feeling so exhausted and my IBD (inflammatory bowel disease) is acting up again. There are some days I am simply in too much pain to work and I feel worthless on those days! (Long pause.) These feelings take me back to my childhood. After my father left, I felt I was of value to my mother only for the work I did. There was no comfort – only many extra tasks, because some days our mother was too depressed to get out of bed and I had to do all the cooking and cleaning. Alone and overworked. Not allowed to spend time with friends. I think of my life today just like my childhood: Only valued for what I can do. Alone and overworked – only eight years old. A little laborer.

Your Inner Process and Attunement
Core fear/longing: _____

Your bodily resonance of her fear or unmet longing: _____

Interpersonal antidote: Find words to describe an interpersonal antidote to the core.

_____

_____

_____

Your Seeding Attachment Intervention

_____

_____

_____

Emily's Inner Process and Attunement

Core fear/longing: Emily identifies the core fear as a harshly negative view of self as of no value and of others as punitive, untrustworthy, and discriminatory. The longing she hears is to have an experience of value and safety. While it is happening at work in her present life and she will return to that, she hears Sahra is now focused on this core experience and unmet need in her childhood.

Resonance: Emily resonates in her own body to how she imagines that fear of worthlessness must feel and she feels small and shaky and like hiding in shame. The sense of longing to be of value, however, feels like a little fire in her belly and she is drawn to Sahra's longing as a spark of life and light.

Interpersonal antidote: She senses in Sahra's story of herself as a little laborer at eight years old, that Sahra feels some indignation that she was treated that way and also some secret respect for that little self. Emily prepares to seed an attachment image of Sahra, receiving care, respect, and comfort.

Emily's Seeding Attachment

Read Emily's response out loud to feel the full impact of the heightened fear and the heightened vision of how, specifically, an interpersonal interaction can soothe or transform this fear.

EMILY: Very difficult to imagine that little laborer at eight years old receiving the respect, safety, and comfort she deserved, isn't it? She never had her mother stepping in to say – oh brave little one, you are so alone and so overworked! This is not fair. You deserve to be a child and to run and play and laugh. You deserve to know you are safe and we will get through our big loss of *Aabo* (her father) together. That beautiful little self, being honored and cared for – you can't imagine that happening back then at all! Is that right?

Your Strengths and Discoveries about Seeding Attachment

_____

_____

_____

Congratulations! If you've done all the workouts in Part 1, you have just completed 61 EFT micro-skills workouts. If you have also done the micro-skills workouts in the online supplement you'll have done 91 in total. Now, with your EFT muscles in shape, you are ready to put it all together in the EFT Tango workouts in Part 2.

Part 2

EFT Tango Workouts

Table of Contents

PART 2.1: INTRODUCING THE EFT TANGO WITH CASE EXAMPLES

The micro-interventions you have been practicing in Part 1 of this book come together in the EFT macro-intervention, known as the EFT Tango. Reference to the therapist macro-intervention as the EFT Tango may sound whimsical or lighthearted at first glance, however, Johnson's metaphorical reference to the macro-intervention of EFT as a series of five (tango) moves is a guide for exquisite attunement for all of therapy and for shaping change events. Just as Argentine tango dancing requires deeply connected attunement and improvisation, the therapeutic change process requires that therapists be attuned moment-to-moment with their clients and with their own inner experience. At the heart of change in EFT is therapists' synchronized attunement with clients through their steps of change.

When a tango dancer knows the five basic tango moves, they can flow creatively between moves. In EFT, when the five moves are integrated into a therapist's way of being, the moves are engaged in an artistic flow. The five moves entail: Reflecting present process; assembling and deepening emotion; shaping engaged encounters; processing the experience of the encounter; and summarizing to integrate and heighten the newly created experience.

While there is no strict linear pattern to follow, there is an organic flow where Move 2 assembly and deepening of emotion flows naturally from Move 1 accurate, empathic reflection of present process. There is also frequently an organic flow from clearly assembled and heightened emotion through Move 2, to shaping, with Move 3, an encounter to express this organized, alive, emotional experience to a significant other, either in the room, or in an individual client's imagination. Move 4 to process and linger with the experience of this engaged encounter, again follows organically, as does Move 5, to integrate and summarize the newly created experience. Repetitions of Moves 2, 3, and 4 are very common. A therapist can repeatedly default to Move 1, reflecting present process, to ground self and the client(s) in the present moment. When present process is clearly reflected, clients feel deeply understood, and there is nonjudgmental coherence in their present-moment story. Move 5 is important at least once in every session to bring together and validate the worth and make coherence of the exploration clients have done.

DOI: 10.4324/9781003242666-2

To introduce the EFT Tango workouts, this section of the book contains descriptions of each move, followed by an EFCT example with Charlie and Hayden, a queer couple who both use they/them pronouns, and an EFIT example with Keiko, a trauma survivor who uses she/her pronouns. Following this are the *EFT Tango Workouts* where you accompany Emily, flowing in attunement between the EFT Tango moves, first with a couple in Part 2.2 and then with an individual client in Part 2.3, to facilitate EFT Stages of client change.

Move 1: Reflecting Present Process

Move 1 reflects and tracks patterns of triggers and action tendencies (the more …the more) optionally adding the emotional impact of this pattern.

The earlier experiential workouts on empathic attuning, reflecting, and validating give you an opportunity to strengthen your *empathic attunement, empathic reflection,* and *validation* muscles. Keep those muscles active and increasingly strong throughout all of EFT! In addition, for Move 1, you will be making many *tracking reflections,* linking within and between dynamics, the inter- and intra-personal. Tracking reflections link trigger and action tendency ("the more… the more…"). The more of a particular external, contextual/interpersonal trigger, the more of the same default response, internally and interpersonally. The clarity of trigger and action tendency offers clients coherence and agency in their emotional dilemmas. They are no longer simply stuck as a person who is not coping well or stuck with a difficult person or an overwhelming circumstance; they are active participants in, as well as victims of, a pattern that can be stabilized and shifted.

Move 1 Reflecting Present Process focuses specifically on forming tracking reflections of observable elements (the more surface elements) of emotion-in-action. We pay specific attention to the surface parts of emotion that can be explicitly observed. The following workouts fine-tune your muscles to identify the surface elements for each client:

What is the cue? (trigger)

What do you do? (action tendency)

Tracking reflections are particularly important for identifying interactional patterns of how inner and outer realities mirror and create each other when clients are in Stage 1. When couple and individual clients stabilize and move into Stages 2 and 3, tracking reflections are "more likely to involve reflecting changes to the negative cycle and the beginning of a new, more positive cycle" (Johnson, 2020, p. 177). For example, in Stage 2, a previously withdrawn partner's shifting experience is tracked as, "Now when you see your partner in distress, you move close to offer comfort."

Emotion-in-action

To dance in attunement with clients, therapists track and reflect the active strategies people are using to survive in their social and relational contexts. Strategies and positions of anxious hyper-activating or avoidant de-activating become self-reinforcing, forming repetitive, increasingly rigid patterns.

In EFCT, these patterns are frequently referred to as cycles or patterns of pursue/demand – defend/withdraw. For example, the more one partner pushes and demands, the more the other defends and shuts down; the more one partner defends and shuts down, the more the other pushes and demands.

In EFIT, the patterns are acknowledged as *best attempt, default strategies,* and repetitive patterns of interacting with others, with self, and with one's socio-cultural context. For example, the more others dismiss and minimize what an individual says, the more the individual may also dismiss their own thoughts and feelings, and the more they dismiss their own thoughts and feelings and longings, the more they experience that others do not listen to them or take them seriously.

Empowering to Discover the Emotional Logic in Survival Strategies

EFT Tango Move 1 workouts help clients to own and recognize their habitual ways of engaging with self and others, when threatened. Recognizing the threatening trigger is often challenging. For example, a therapist may be thinking, "This client is angry – and what triggers their anger is that they are overwhelmed." But "being overwhelmed" is not an interpersonal trigger. The therapist can identify the action tendency – to have angry outbursts – but not have identified the trigger for the angry reactions. After they can identify *when* a client gets angry (for example, when demands are made of them), then they have named the trigger. Making the link between triggers and reflexive action responses and patterns frequently becomes an empowering discovery process for clients. Naming, "This is what I do in reaction to that threatening cue," gives a client a sense of agency, as in, "I am an actor in my drama, not a passive recipient of other's antics." This opens the door to awareness and empowerment to find new meanings, new feelings, and new action tendencies.

To do Move 1, EFT therapists ask themselves:

1. Am I attuned to the threatening cue the client is experiencing? For example, in EFCT, am I aware that what triggered the partner was likely their partner's looking away or saying nothing in reply? In EFIT, can I identify the external or interpersonal trigger that sets the pattern of self-protection or isolation in motion?
2. What does the client reflexively do in the face of a threatening cue? Does a partner fire up in exasperation if their partner is silent or looks away as they speak animatedly about something? Is an individual client triggered to respond in self-defeating ways, such as giving to others to the point of burnout, across a series of relationships (family and social relationships) in response to an experience of abandonment?

Finding the links between cues and action tendencies keeps the attachment/relational frame alive. Emotion is about self and system.

EFCT Example of Tango Move 1, Reflecting Present Process

So Charlie, the more Hayden complains about the messy house, the more you sink into depression and loneliness, and pull away in a quiet funk. And Hayden, the more Charlie pulls away into what you call a "seething sulk," the more irritated and annoyed you become. Each of you is alone and miserable, feeling unwanted and lonely.

EFIT Example of Tango Move 1, Reflecting Present Process

Keiko, I hear the prison you feel trapped in: Seeing others acting pleasant and friendly on the surface, sends you into a cascade of suspicion and self-doubts. You say there is something about their "niceness" that feels disingenuous and not to be trusted. These others include your uncle, your colleagues, and guys with whom you have had just one date. "I don't trust anyone," you say. You doubt that others, especially the very friendly and nice ones, like you or trust you, and in fact, you say, "I can't trust myself either to have any competence or likeability!" You live in a revolving-door prison of keeping a safe distance from others and staying safely numb and distanced from your own self-doubts and fears.

Move 2: Assembling and Deepening Emotion

The goals of Tango Move 2 are: (1) to discover the elements of emotion; (2) to assemble, link, and distill them into a coherent whole; and (3) to deepen that whole *or* core emotion into an alive, vivid experience where new depths, edges, and felt shifts of emotional experiencing and previously implicit feelings and meanings emerge. This can be described as 3 D's (discover, distill, and deepen):

1. **Discover** elements of emotion, evoking unexpressed, and hidden elements.
2. **Distill** (link, assemble, expand, and distill) into a coherent whole.
3. **Deepen** and bring to life.

Micro-Interventions Used in Move 2

Empathic attunement explicitly focuses on the active, rapid unfolding **elements** of emotion.

Evocative responses and questions to invite more granularity and specificity of the different elements of the active process of emotion. Evocative questions for specific elements of emotion are below.

Empathic tracking reflections to link different elements of emotion together, into a coherent whole of core emotion.

Heightening with RISSSSSC manner to expand elements of emotion as they are being assembled and to savor and deepen the newly simplified whole, in the context of working models of self, other, and the social-cultural context.

Conjectures are focused on staying very close to the client's experience, yet slightly on the leading edge of attachment emotional experience.

Evocative Questions toward Specific Elements of Emotion

As new elements of emotion are being evoked, they can be linked to an element already identified, as exemplified below:

To evoke the **trigger:** *When* do you find yourself doing that (action tendency) or *When* do you tell yourself that or when do you make that distressing meaning?

To evoke the **sense of threat**: How does this information, this look, this gesture, etc. (name the trigger), land with you, impact you? Touch you?

To evoke **bodily arousal**: Where in your body... what happens inside when your jaw tightens (to evoke more bodily arousal), what else happens inside? When you take that to mean _____ (meaning making), how does your body respond?

To evoke the **meaning** being made, what does that (trigger) say to you? What meaning do you make of (the trigger)? How do you make sense of that?

To evoke the **action tendency** or impulse or reactive emotion: What do you feel like doing, or typically do when _____?

General Evocative Questions

General questions can also be used to explore present-moment experiences.

Examples: What is happening for you as _____? What is it like to notice _____?

Link general questions to elements already identified. Repeating a specific element makes the question more evocative and pulls for more engagement from the client. For example: What is it like to notice how you quickly throw up your hands in defeat when you say with all this tension in your jaw, "Injustice. This wasn't right!"?

Deepening with RISSSSSC

RISSSSSC is an acronym for: **R**epetition, **I**mages, **S**imple, **S**oft, **S**low, **S**pecific, **S**omatic, **C**lient's words. Using a RISSSSSC manner to deepen (aka heighten) is essentially staying close to clients' experience – mirroring/bringing alive their experience with repetition, using evocative images, especially the ones they come up with on their own, in a simple, soft, slow manner, with specific words, reflecting somatic signals (verbal and non-verbal), and repeating clients' words. Softness is not always the tone. Most important is to slow down to match the client's core emotional intensity. Heightening with RISSSSSC is an integral part of how EFT interventions are done. It is how elements of emotion are expanded as they are being assembled and how the newly simplified whole/core emotion is savored and heightened/deepened.

RISSSSSC manner is a very important part of the two main tasks of Tango Move 2 assembly and deepening/heightening:

1. Assemble (link together) the core elements of emotion. This creates a sense of completeness and clarity about experience. Using the RISSSSSC manner, elements of emotion are expanded as they are being assembled and linked together.
2. Deepen/Heighten each element as they are being assembled. Savoring and heightening the newly coherent whole opens doors to further discovery.

EFCT Example of Tango Move 2 Assembly and Deepening
(elements of emotion in parentheses)

Therapist: Charlie, help me understand what Hayden's pleas for you to pay more attention to picking up after yourself and keeping the house tidier (trigger) say to you (evoking meaning of the trigger).

Charlie: That Hayden is totally fed up with me, doesn't understand me, will never accept me for who I am.

Having evoked the meaning, the therapist links elements of emotion into a coherent whole.

Therapist: Hayden comes home, and before you hear they are happy to see you, you see that look on Hayden's face (trigger), like just before the storm begins – a look that says, "You are about to hear a tirade of reasons why I cannot accept you," (meaning) and you find yourself freezing and going numb (body arousal; linking trigger, meaning, and bodily response).

Charlie: Yes, that look (trigger) is all it takes! On the outside, I freeze and can't seem to move (action tendency), but inside, my stomach seizes into a knot that says, "You're doomed. Hayden has already given up on you!"

One more Move 2, this time, to deepen the core, underlying attachment fear.

Therapist: Under your frozen exterior is a panicked knot in your gut trembling with fear that Hayden has already given up on you, and you freeze, can't even move, so afraid that Hayden is already judging you as unacceptable!

EFIT Example of Tango Move 2 Assembly and Deepening
(elements of emotion in parentheses)
Therapist: Keiko, your stomach churns (body arousal) with this painful sense of how unjust it is (meaning) that your abusive uncle smiles and acts pleasant and kind, when behind your back he has done these subtle, hurtful things to you (trigger). Inside, your stomach churns and the pain becomes rage, and you want to find a safe way to express this rage (action tendency), yes?

Move 3: Shaping Engaged Encounters

The goal of Move 3 is to shape an engaged encounter that is relevant to the emotion that is being assembled and deepened. Encounters are preceded by different degrees of emotion assembly and are chosen for different functions, depending on where clients are in the steps and stages of the EFT change process. The different functions of encounters are to help clients: own action tendencies and stuck positions and habitual patterns; access or deepen core emotion; share newly accessed core emotion in a clear message; make a specific request to meet an attachment need emerging from core emotion; and revisit and celebrate newly shaped interpersonal connection.

Engaged Encounters are shaped in the following manner with various micro-interventions. The process can be denoted by the acronym SHAPE:

Sharpen the core, assembled message to be shared. Use empathic tracking reflections of what was discovered, distilled, and deepened with Move 2.

Heighten the emotional experience of the message, repeating key elements of emotion, mirroring and slightly heightening with RISSSSSC. Using proxy voice also heightens clients' present-moment experiencing.

Anticipate the experience of disclosing and establish sufficient safety from the listener with evocative responses and questions, repetition, and possibly seeding attachment.

Present: Repeat the message and direct the client to **Present** it.

Engage: Refocus, redirect, and slice risks thinner, when needed.

EFCT Example of Move 3 Shaping Engaged Encounter

Sharpen the message: Charlie, you are saying Hayden is your most important person, but you do find yourself pulling away from what you call the "unpredictable tirades" that sound to you like you are not even wanted anymore. You are pulling away, getting quiet, and losing motivation to pick up after yourself, when inside, you are fearing that Hayden is fed up with you!

Heighten the message (in proxy voice): So afraid you are fed up with me, that I do get quiet, pull inside myself, and let the clutter build up, feeling overwhelmed and helpless to regain your approval.

Anticipate sharing the message: Can you look at Hayden in front of you and can you imagine sharing this message, telling Hayden that, "Yes, I am pulling away and letting clutter build up, when inside I am terrified that I have no way to ever regain your approval again?" And Hayden, can you listen to Charlie share this with you? (Hayden nods, "Of course!")

Direct to **Present the message**: Can you share this with Hayden now – share how you know you are pulling away and letting clutter build up, getting overwhelmed and terrified it is too late to regain Hayden's approval?

Engage: If Charlie hesitates and says, "I don't think I can do that," or, "I already said it," the therapist can be transparent: I know it feels awkward, but I'd really like each of you to have this experience of you turning to Hayden and sharing that your pulling away and letting clutter build up is how you are coping with this terror that you have no hope anymore of gaining Hayden's approval. Can you try it, please?

If Charlie says, "I really don't want to admit that I do this," the therapist can slice the message more thinly to make it manageable: I hear it is embarrassing. Can you turn to Hayden and share that for now it's just too hard to share that you deal with your fear of having lost Hayden's approval by pulling away and letting clutter build up?

EFIT Example of Move 3 Shaping Engaged Encounter

Sharpen the message: Keiko, I am wondering if we can shape a message from this rage in your churning stomach that says to your uncle, "What you did to me was wrong! You are cruel and unjust, and I still hurt after all these years!"

Heighten the message (in proxy voice): So wrong. You did it with a cunning, nasty smile and I am enraged with you! I hold you entirely responsible for damaging my childhood!

Anticipate sharing the message: Can you picture your uncle just now? Just notice what comes up inside for you to picture him? What does he look like? Does he say anything? Do you feel safe to close your eyes and imagine he was here to listen to a very important message from you? What else might you need to make it safe to speak to an image of your uncle, as you see him just now? If she needs to tell him she does not want to hear back from an image of him, the therapist will support her to express that limit directly to her imaginal uncle, such as, "I'm going to say my piece to you, and I do not want to hear anything back from you!"

Direct to **Present the message**: Can you tell him now, about the rage in your stomach? About how what he did was totally wrong and how you hold him responsible?

Engage: If Keiko gets distracted or frightened, the therapist grounds her with their presence and with the rage in her churning stomach. The therapist can *slice the message thinner* if Keiko needs them to: Tell him for now then, "I'm not ready to talk with this image of you, but I have a lot to say, and I'll call you back in my imagination when I am ready to do so."

Move 4: Processing Engaged Encounters

EFT therapists process and savor the new moment of interpersonal contact with Move 4. Present-moment experience is heightened by slowing down to repeat the message shared before eliciting from the discloser how it was to share the message and with the recipient how it was to receive this message. This repetition or *mining the moment* to deepen, to make the most of it, is a hallmark of two factors shown to lead to a change in EFT: Increasing depth of emotional experience and affiliative interactions. Repeating the core message that was shared and anything the therapist observed in the disclosure helps to retain focus and deepen the level of emotional experience.

An example of Move 4 processing with a discloser: How was it to turn to your partner, your voice got very quiet and you looked down, as you told your partner, "It is true, I do get louder and louder when your look tells me you don't even care about me." What was that like for you as you shared that with your partner?

An example of Move 4 processing with the recipient: I noticed as your partner shared that she does get louder and louder towards you when you shrug your shoulders or give her a look that tells her you don't care, that you reached out and put your hand on her leg. What is happening inside for you as you hear this and reach out to touch her?

Micro-interventions used in Move 4 include reflection, repetition, evocative questions, heightening, and catching bullets if needed.

EFCT Example of Move 4, Processing an Engaged Encounter

How was it Charlie, to look right at Hayden and to say, "It's true, I do pull away and let clutter build up. I just get overwhelmed and give up – so afraid you'll never give me another chance and worry I am losing you?" And Hayden, what happens inside you as Charlie looks right at you and says, "It is true – I do pull away and let clutter build up when inside the fear of losing you is overwhelming and the chance of regaining your favor seems impossible?" What is it like for you to hear this from Charlie?

EFIT Example of Move 4, Processing an Engaged Encounter

Keiko, you just took an enormous risk to look straight at this image of your old uncle and tell him how badly he hurt you and how wrong and unacceptable it was! How was it to speak so clearly to him from the rage in your churning stomach? (Pause to give Keiko time to respond.) And how do you imagine your uncle to be responding just now? What more do you want to say in response?

Move 5: Integration and Validation

The goal of Move 5 is to integrate, validate, and summarize. It can be used in the midst of sessions and at the end of sessions, such as, "Today, Charlie, you shared so clearly with Hayden what happens inside of you when you are letting clutter build up, instead of pulling away and getting quiet as you do in your typical pattern. And you, Hayden, welcomed Charlie and you were touched, instead of getting louder and unhappy with them."

With Move 5 a therapist summarizes and validates a change event or a new moment of contact, integrating and heightening the corrective emotional experience of new moments of engaged contact just created between two individuals. The summary, validation, and integration of Move 5 often feel like a celebration, focusing on positive affect and emotional balance. During stabilization, it is useful to draw the contrast between the old cycle or pattern and the new moves they are taking, or even the ways they are now able to stop the old pattern and talk about what they are doing and the fears driving them. In Stages 2 and 3, Move 5 also includes highlighting the new moves and emerging changes.

Micro-interventions for Move 5 include empathic tracking reflections of changes and change events, heightening, and summarizing.

EFCT Example of Move 5 Integration and Validation

You have come a long way together in recognizing and stopping your automatic push–pull dance. Now, when Charlie pulls away and becomes quiet, you, Hayden, know Charlie's messes and pulling away are signs of their being overwhelmed and frightened of losing your favor and feeling powerless to regain your acceptance. And Charlie, you don't pull away so much anymore, now that you get that Hayden's complaints are not meant to reject and discard you but are rather code for their fears that you have stopped caring about your relationship. Seeing each other differently, as frightened, not mean or uncaring, the push–pull pattern is slowing way down and when it occurs, you are often able to stop it and discuss what is happening between you and name the fears you are fighting in the background.

EFIT Example of Move 5 Integration and Validation

The risks you have taken, Keiko, seem to be having an enormous impact in loosening the bars of your revolving-door prison, where the more you distanced from others who all seemed unsafe and manipulative, the more you distanced from your own inner experience and trust in yourself. You trusted our conversations enough to discover words for your very real inner rage at the ones who have abused you. You listened to your own inner sense enough to risk telling your imaginal uncle how unjust his treatment of you was. You are beginning to experience that all others may not be mean and manipulative and not-to-be-trusted. You are beginning to move closer to me and to your own inner experience, and to have a strong, clear message to tell another, "You stole my sense of my own goodness, and I am going to get it back!"

Moves and Micro-Skills in the EFT Tango

Move 1 Reflecting and Tracking Processes and Patterns

Empathic attunement, reflection, tracking patterns of triggers, and action tendencies (linking within and between, inter and intra).

Move 2 Assembly and Deepening

Evocative Responses and Questions to invite more granularity and specificity of the different elements of the active process of emotion.
Empathic tracking reflections to link different elements of emotion together.
Heightening to deepen core emotion and working models of self and other and the social-cultural context.

Tango Move 3 SHAPE Encounters (aka enactments; affiliative interactions)

S Sharpen message (use reflection and RISSSSSC).
H Heighten (with RISSSSSC).
A Anticipate sharing and receiving (sometimes *seeding attachment*).
P Direct to Present (*slice thinner* if needed).
E Engage (redirect, refocus).

Tango Move 4 Processing Encounters

Evocative questions, reflecting, heightening, and *catching bullets* if needed.

Tango Move 5 Integration and Validation

Summarize and integrate with empathic tracking reflections, validation, heightening, and summarizing.

PART 2.2: EFCT TANGO WORKOUTS WITH MEI-LING AND AKI

The series of workouts that follow provide you with opportunities to apply all the EFT micro-interventions, also known as micro-skills, in the EFT macro-intervention, the EFT Tango. You have an opportunity to practice the moves of the tango, alongside Emily with a couple, Mei-Ling and Aki. Mei-Ling, born in Singapore, and her husband Aki, born in Japan, both immigrated with their parents to North America as toddlers. They have been married for 11 years. A pattern of emotional distancing is intensifying between them, with Mei-Ling getting progressively more frustrated with Aki and Aki throwing up his hands in futility.

A narrative preview of the therapeutic steps of change that you can facilitate with Mei-Ling and Aki through the following 20 EFT Tango workouts is available in Part 2.2 Support Material on-line (at routledge.com/9781032151311). Each workout ends with space for you to identify your strengths in forming that particular EFT Tango move and anything you may have discovered from Emily's response that you want to integrate into your style.

EFCT Tango Workout 1: Move 1, Reflecting Present Process

For Move 1 workouts, stick to the observable triggers and reactions even though you will undoubtedly intuit affective experience and be tempted to conjecture many of the internally experienced elements of emotion that are on the leading edge of what the client has expressed. The goal here is to fine-tune your ability to distinguish the initial trigger and behavioral response elements of emotion from the greater depths (bodily, meaning-making, emotion words) that are hinted at on the leading edge. Helping clients to identify, "This what triggers me and this is how I respond" is part of how we create the validating, coherent, empowering, and non-pathologizing experience of secure attachment. To workout your EFT muscles, you are encouraged to add a general summary of the affective tone only after you link the triggers and action tendencies, such as what each one does when feeling lonely and miserable as they both are.

How to Do Move 1 Reflecting Present Process

1. Attune to the pattern of trigger and action tendency and to the emotional impact of this pattern.
2. Resonate – in your own body with:
   a. the triggering experience (likely the partner's action tendency) and
   b. how the client responds (action tendency).
   If you have not yet identified the trigger and the action tendency, continue to be curious to discover the trigger the client perceives as threatening or challenging and the client's action tendency. Pure empathy for how difficult a situation may be for a client without understanding *what triggers them and how they are responding to the threatening cue is not enough. We are collaborating with clients to identify their strategies/patterns. It is empowering for clients to explore the patterns of how they are engaging with life – with self, with others, and with the context of their experience.*

3. Find words and use the client's words to formulate the link between trigger and action impulse. "The more... the more..."
4. Check for confirmation that your words match the client's experience. Verbally ("Yes?") or non-verbally (with tentativeness through voice inflection) invite the client to confirm, adjust or correct your words (communicated empathic understanding).

Read the couple's comments below out loud.

Mei-Ling: (Shrill voice) Why don't you ever make traditional soup when I am sick or working evenings!? You never help out with household responsibilities anymore or with the children's schoolwork! I am alone in this relationship. I have to take responsibility for everything!! Why don't you carry your share of responsibility?

Aki: (Shrugs, throws up hands, looks at therapist.) See what I have to put up with? I don't understand why this is such a big deal. My father didn't do anything at home and my mom didn't complain. I know we have agreed to share domestic tasks, however, my job is much more demanding than yours, and I don't see what's wrong for you to pick up more when I am too busy to worry about dishes.

Following the prompts below create your own Move 1 reflecting present process.
Your Inner Process and Attunement

Most poignant emotional impact communicated by Mei-Ling: _____

Most poignant emotional impact communicated by Aki: _____

Identify what Mei-Ling does that is a threat to Aki: _____

Identify what Aki does that is a threat to Mei-Ling: _____

Your bodily experience as you resonate with this pattern (of the more... the more...):

_____

Your Move 1 Reflection of Present Process

Using behavioral, nonjudgmental words (e.g. get louder, turn away) track how they are triggered by each other. Formulate the link ("the more...the more") between triggers and responses (optionally adding emotional impact on each partner):

_____

_____

Compare your responses with Emily's responses below. Your responses may be very different from Emily's and that is ok.
Emily's Inner Process and Attunement

The most poignant emotional impact that Emily attunes to with Mei-Ling is a desperate call for response in a caring, nourishing way as with traditional soup. With Aki, she is struck by his frustrated, automatic, pull-away pattern. She picks up a sense of futility and aloneness in both partners.

Emily identifies the triggers and responses unfolding before her.

<u>What Mei-Ling does that threatens Aki:</u> She lists with a shrill voice what Aki does not do and how she feels alone! Hearing her complaint of feeling alone is likely a trigger for Aki.

<u>What Aki does that is a threat to Mei-Ling:</u> He shrugs and turns away and says he is *putting up* with Mei-Ling's comments.

<u>Emily's bodily experience as she resonates with this pattern</u>: She feels an emptiness in her own stomach as she sees Mei-Ling triggered by Aki's shrug and comment about putting up with her message. She feels a solid block, like a protective shield, in her heart as she sees Aki triggered by Mei-Ling's shrill voice as she lists what he doesn't do and how alone she feels.

To form a Move 1 reflection of the present process, Emily wants to avoid words like *complaining, shrieking,* and *nonchalance* because she thinks those words will convey judgment and she knows hearing judgment is code for attachment panic on both parts. She also wants to avoid conjecturing and instead simply reflect on the drama unfolding in the moment, because she knows this will offer the couple a refreshing reframe of two people accusing each other.

Emily's Move 1 Reflection of Present Process

Seems the louder and more insistent you, Mei-Ling, become, about how you want more from Aki, the more you, Aki, shrug and turn away… It sounds, Mei-Ling, like you have a very important message you want Aki to hear. Something about traditional soup from Aki means a lot to you. And Aki, you shrug your shoulders, and throw up your hands, like you don't know what to do. The louder you, Mei-Ling, get, the more you, Aki, turn away and the more you, Aki, turn away, the louder, you, Mei-Ling, become, yes? Round and round it goes with each of you frustrated and alone.

Your Strengths and Discoveries about Move 1

_____

_____

EFCT Tango Workout 2: Move 2 Workout to Assemble Emotional Experience

How to Do Move 2 Assembly

Tracking explicit elements of emotion, expanding elements, and evoking hidden elements of emotion.

1. Identify *an emotional/cultural handle* that strikes you as the salient part of the message, to expand.
2. Repeat it aloud and get the feel of this *emotional handle* in your own body.
3. Notice the explicit elements of emotion the client is conveying; consider:

   - What is the cue/trigger that signals a threat?
   - What are the somatic reactions (facial or bodily movements)?
   - What is the client saying about the meanings they are making?

> - What are the client's action tendencies?
> - What elements are missing or are very general and you will want to evoke, expand, or deepen?
>
> 4. Repeat the elements in a vivid, specific manner, matching the client's emotional tone. Then, make a clear invitation to expand on a specific hidden element or to invite more specific exploration of a vaguely stated element, such as, "Tell me more about ___."

Read the couple's comments below out loud.

AKI: It's been a hard week. Mei-Ling was sick and (shrugs his shoulders) she says I am the worst husband ever.

MEI-LING: (Shrill voice) There is that clued-out, innocent look again! It's like he hears nothing, no matter how desperately I try to get his attention! (Tension in her face and in her hands.)

Your Inner Process and Attunement

What explicit elements of Mei-Ling's emotional experience has she expressed (trigger perceived as threatening, bodily arousal, meaning-making, action tendency)? _____

_____

What hint of attachment panic (more meaning) do you hear? _____

Your Move 2 Assembly

Link these elements together in a Move 2 assembly: _____

_____

What elements of emotion do you want to expand or evoke? _____
Create some Move 2 evocative responses or questions to evoke more:

_____

_____

Emily's Inner Process and Attunement

Emily notes the elements of emotion that Mei-Ling has already shared.
<u>Perceived threatening cue/trigger</u>: A look on Aki's face; his shrug.
<u>Body</u>: Tense.
<u>Meaning</u>: He doesn't hear me.
<u>Action tendency</u>: She gets louder; lists what Aki has not done,
<u>Hints of attachment panic</u> (more meaning): "I can't reach him / get him to notice me / to respond when I need him."

Emily's Move 2 Assembly
(Linking elements Mei-Ling expressed.) So, you see a look on Aki's face (*cue*) and you automatically get louder and louder (*action tendency, body voice*). You tell yourself that look means he is not hearing you (*meaning*) and you become desperate to reach him *(hint of attachment panic)*.
(To elicit more about Mei-Ling's meaning-making and bodily arousal.) Can you tell me more about what his look says to you?
(To evoke more about the poignant attachment image and cultural handle.) Can you say more about what Aki cooking traditional soup when you are sick means to you?
(To elicit more bodily arousal.) You speak of desperately trying to get his attention. Can you tell me more about how that sense of desperateness feels in your body?

Your Strengths and Discoveries about Move 2 Assembly

_____

_____

EFCT Tango Workout 3: Move 2 to Deepen Emotional Experience

How to Do Move 2 to Deepen Emotional Engagement

1. Identify an *emotional handle* that captures the *emotion-story* assembled thus far. The emotional handle can be bodily movements, images, or poignant phrases.
2. Resonate with how this emotional handle feels in your own body.
3. Slowly and simply repeat the assembled *emotion-story*, optionally in proxy voice. Resist inferences and conjectures. Matching the client's emotional tone is likely to evoke a slightly deeper level than what the client has conveyed.

This newly coherent, deepened, simplified whole, is likely to prime the client for an encounter.

Read Emily's Move 2 evocative questions and Mei-Ling's responses below out loud.

EMILY: (To elicit more about the meaning Mei-Ling is making.) Can you tell me more about what that look says to you?

MEI-LING: (In response to her sense that Aki is not listening.) That, he doesn't care and that he is totally fine with me carrying all the responsibilities!

EMILY: (To elicit more about her bodily arousal.) When you sense he is not hearing you, you said you become desperate to reach him, can you tell me more about how that sense of desperateness feels in your body?

MEI-LING: It's a big cavern in me. My heart is hollow, my stomach is empty and I am all alone – isolated a cold, barren wasteland.

Following the prompts below create your own Move 2 deepening response that links Mei-Ling's core emotion to her ownership of her action tendency to get loud and complain about Aki.

Your Inner Process and Attunement

Choose an *emotional* handle from Mei-Ling's expression above. _____

Note your bodily resonance, so that when you speak, you are likely to evoke a slightly deeper level than what the client has conveyed. _____

Your Move 2 Deepening *with RISSSSSC*

Repeat the elements of emotion as conveyed in this image, resisting conjectures; make explicit the link between trigger and action tendency:

_____

_____

Slowly and simply say the newly coherent simplified whole aloud, matching Mei-Ling's emotional tone.

Notice how this can make sense of her action tendency and prepare her for a Stage 1 engaged encounter, to own her action tendency as linked to her underlying fear.

Emily's Inner Process and Attunement

Emily is struck by these *emotional handles* from Mei-Ling: all alone; a hollow cavern in my body; alone in a cold, barren wasteland!

As she resonates with a sense of a hollow cavern in the core of her own body, and the terror of being isolated in a wasteland with no one in sight, she is struck with realizing this is what Mei-Ling is feeling when her voice increases in volume and she complains about Aki.

Emily's Move 2 Deepening with RISSSSSC

You see a look on Aki's face that to you says, "Oh, oh, he's not hearing me, maybe he doesn't care," and you feel hollow, empty, all alone without him, isolated in a cold desolate wasteland and in your desperation to reach him and get him to respond to you, your voice gets louder and louder, and you get more and more frustrated with him, yes?

Your Strengths and Discoveries about Deepening in Move 2

_____

_____

EFCT Tango Workout 4: Move 3 Shaping an Engaged Encounter to Own Action Tendency

How to Do Move 3 Shaping Encounters

Workouts for EFT Tango Move 3: SHAPE an Engaged Encounter

S Sharpen message (use reflection)

H Heighten (with repetition)

> **A Anticipate** sharing and receiving (sometimes *seeding attachment*)
> **P** Direct to **Present** (*slice thinner* if needed)
> **E Engage** (redirect, refocus, *catch bullets*) *if needed*

Following the prompts below, SHAPE an engaged encounter with Tango Move 3 to help Mei-Ling disclose what was deepened in the previous workout.

Insert your responses after each prompt, comparing with Emily's as you go, to discover anything you may want to integrate into your EFT *manner of shaping engaged encounters*. Emily's responses are immediately after the space for you to insert your response, so you may wish to place a piece of paper over her response, so you can make your response without interference. Your responses may be very different from Emily's and that is ok. The important thing is that you find a way to sharpen, heighten, anticipate, direct presentation of the message, and re-engage when needed.

Your Sharpening
With an empathic tracking reflection, repeat the core message that was discovered, distilled, and deepened for Mei-Ling with Move 2. Optionally, use proxy voice: _____
_____
_____

Emily's Sharpening
I'd like to help you shape a message to share with Aki to tell him, that, "Yes, my voice does get loud and shrill when I see that look on your face that tells me you are not hearing me. I am alone, afraid you don't care. My loud voice comes from within a cold empty place where I cannot find you anywhere. Cannot get you to respond to me or show that you care! My plea for that simple bowl of soup is my call to show me you care, but my call does get loud and full of annoyance at him."

Your Heightening
Repeating key elements of emotion, mirroring and slightly heightening with RISSSSSC; using proxy voice also heightens preset-moment experiencing: _____
_____
_____

Emily's Heightening
A barren wilderness cold, empty, all alone. Calling loud and louder to get him to see me. To get him to hear me! To get him to move and show he cares!

Your Anticipation
Help Aki to anticipate sharing the message. Establish sufficient safety with Aki, with evocative responses, questions, and repetition. _____
_____

Emily's Anticipation

Can you look at Aki just now and imagine sharing this message with him – telling him how you recognize you do get louder and louder when you see a look on his face that says to you he doesn't really care, that tells you he is leaving you alone; that you do start getting louder and louder to get him to hear you and respond to you?

Aki, can you listen to Mei-Ling as she shares with you, how she knows she does get louder and louder from her panic of feeling alone – sensing that perhaps you don't care and don't mind leaving her alone with all the responsibilities? Is it ok to let her share with you the panic that is going on inside when she gets loud with you?

Your Directing to <u>Present</u>

Repeat the message and direct the client to Present it. (Assuming Aki has confirmed he is ready to hear from her.) _____

_____

Emily's Directing to <u>Present</u>

Mei-Ling, can you please tell Aki, how you know your voice gets louder and louder when you see the look he just gave you – when you see the look that says to you – "I'm alone, maybe he doesn't even care, so I call after him with a louder and louder voice to get a response." Can you share this with him?

Your Engaging

Imagine Mei-Ling is reluctant to share, saying, "He already knows." How can you re-engage her and slice the request thinner if needed? _____

_____

Emily's Engaging

Option 1: (Transparency to engage Mei-Ling.) It is not easy to do this, I realize. It takes a lot of courage, but I'd like you to have the experience of letting Aki hear directly from you that you are aware that you do get louder and louder when you see his look that tells you he is not really there with you. Can you risk it please?

Option 2: (Transparency to engage Mei-Ling.) I recognize this is difficult to do. He has heard you tell me, but I'd like you to have the experience of turning to him and telling him yourself. He did say he is willing to hear this from you just now. Can you see what is it like to tell him, please?

Option 3: If Mei-Ling says, "No, I will not tell him… I am too angry! He's likely just to shrug his shoulders again with that innocent look!" (Slicing it thinner, to engage Mei-Ling.) What a big chance you would be taking – when you anticipate him shrugging you off! That makes sense – too big a risk. Can you tell him now then, "It's too hard to tell you. I'm too angry. Too afraid you'll shrug me off"?

Your Strengths and Discoveries about Move 3

_____

_____

EFCT Tango Workout 5: Move 4 Processing an Engaged Encounter

> **How to Do Move 4 to Process Encounters**
>
> An effective way to do Move 4 is to:
>
> • Repeat the core of the message that was disclosed, using the client's words and non-verbals, such as eye contact, bodily movements, and voice change.
> • Ask the discloser to describe their experience of sharing this message.
> • Repeat the keywords and non-verbals again and elicit the receiver's felt experience in receiving the message.
>
> Reflections and evocative questions are key micro-skills used in Move 4, along with validation and heightening.

Read Mei-Ling's following encounter, aloud, tuning in as well to how Aki may be feeling as he receives this message.

MEI-LING: Yes, I do come at you loud and aggressive, I do. I see that look on your face or see you shrug your shoulders and I'm filled rage – how can you leave me alone – how can you not care – I feel like you don't even see me and that I am all alone! (Pausing, tearing up; Aki reaches out and places his hand on her leg.) I just get frantic! (Her voice becomes quieter and a slight smile crosses her face.) It's almost like maybe if I yell enough you'll wake up and come to life and prove to me that you care!

Following the prompts below, form Tango Move 4 processing first with Mei-Ling, the discloser and then with Aki, the recipient.

Your Move 4 Responses to Mei-Ling and Aki

After Mei-Ling's engaged encounter with Aki, identify how you will savor and process this experience of the encounter. Experiment with repeating the message shared and any non-verbals you imagine from either partner:

1. Check with her how it was to share: _____

_____

2. Evoke Aki's internal experience as he received this disclosure from Mei-Ling: _____

_____

_____

Emily's Move 4 Response to Mei-Ling

Mei-Ling, how was it to look at Aki and tell him you know your voice gets very loud and you are filled with rage when you take his look and his shrugged shoulders to mean he doesn't care about you? You told him that in fact your high volume is code for trying to get him to prove he cares about you and he placed his hand on your leg. It almost seems like your voice quieted a little as you shared and he touched you. How is it to be sharing this with him?

MEI-LING: (Smiling and hanging her head.) I felt kind of silly sharing it because he already heard me tell you and it is embarrassing to admit I can be a shrieking monster! (Looking up.) But it helped me actually – to see I'm not just a shrieking monster – I am trying to move him into action! I want him to prove to me that he does care!

Emily's Move 4 Response to Aki

Aki, I noticed when Mei-Ling shared with you that she knows she gets loud and aggressive when she sees a certain look on your face or sees you shrug your shoulders that you moved in and put your hand on her leg. What happens inside of you as you move close to hear, hearing her make sense of her loud voice coming from a desperate place of wondering if you care or even see her?

AKI: I'm shocked and relieved actually – It's a relief to hear Mei-Ling recognize she gets loud and aggressive, but it's a real shock to know she thinks I don't see her or don't care! I see her, I feel her, I hear her all the time. I just get frozen because I miss the mark most of the time!

Your Strengths and Discoveries about Move 4

_____

_____

Moves 2 and 3 to Help Aki Own His Action Tendency

Imagine Emily also does the Tango Move 2 assembly with Aki, to help him own his action tendency to turn away or to throw up his hands and shrug his shoulders and do nothing. Picture Emily assembling and deepening Aki's ownership of his action tendency to shrug his shoulders and sometimes walk away, in reaction to Mei-Ling's cries for him to respond. After this assembly and deepening, imagine hearing Emily shape a Move 3 encounter for Aki to disclose to Mei-Ling that when he hears a shrill tone of Mei-Ling's voice (trigger of attachment threat for him), he hears she is disappointed with him (his meaning) and he can no longer hear her words, but that his ears shut down and he simply goes numb and wants to get away from hearing how disappointed she is with him (action tendency). Imagine Aki discloses to Mei-Ling:

I do try to get away from the sound of your voice being disappointed with me. All I hear is that I am a disappointment to you and I can't even hear your words. I just freeze, shrug my shoulders, or tell you to stop talking. I can't bear it.

Move 4 to Process with Each Partner

Visualize that as Emily does Move 4 with each partner, Aki expresses relief to be sharing this with Mei-Ling. Mei-Ling also expresses relief to hear him owning that he does shrug his shoulders and tell her to stop talking, however, she is very shocked and nearly disbelieving that he freezes and gets flooded hearing that she is disappointed in him. She has had no idea what was happening inside for him when he shrugged his shoulders or turned away. She has had no sense that she was having any impact on him at all. This is too much for her to take in, and in her shock and disbelief, she becomes reactive.

Read aloud the following response from Mei-Ling to Aki's disclosure. Resonate with how you would feel if you were Aki, hearing this.

MEI-LING: I am so relieved to hear you admit that you shrug your shoulders or tell me to stop, but (her voice quickens and becomes louder) I can't believe you freeze and get flooded when you hear I am disappointed! I can't trust that you'd even care if you did disappoint me. You say those horrible things like, "This is just a functional relationship, where we each have a job to do."

EFCT Tango Workout 6: Catching a Bullet in Move 4 Processing of an Engaged Encounter

Here in Tango Move 4, Emily hears a small bullet to catch or at least some disorientation to validate.

Follow the formula for catching bullets in response to Mei-Ling's reaction. The goal is to catch a bullet when the receiving partner becomes reactive, in a way that maintains focus on this new experience of contact.
    1. Interrupt Mei-Ling with validation: _____
    2. Reflect present process/what just happened, without judgment, in neutral, behavioral terms:

_____

    3. Reframe the reactivity by conjecturing at confusion, disorientation, or disbelief: _____

_____

    4. Validate the attachment intention: _____
    5. Confirm with Mei-Ling: _____
    6. Refocus: _____

Emily's attempt to catch the bullet and validate Mei-Ling in Move 4

1. Interrupt: Mei-Ling, may I step in, please?
2. Reflect in neutral terms, what just happened: Initially you say you are so relieved to hear Aki acknowledge that he does shrug his shoulders and tell you to stop, but then you find it almost unbelievable that it actually bothers him to hear that you are disappointed in him, and before you know it, you remind him of hurtful things he says.
3. Reframe, conjecture at her disbelief, her fear of trusting, and her disorientation: You don't see that side of him and you can't trust, yet, that he cares about not letting you down.
4. Validate: It is so new and so difficult to believe that he hears he is disappointing you and that he can't bear to hear that. Too risky to believe, yet, that Aki does not like to let you down?
5. Confirm: Am I understanding? (Pause for Mei-Ling's response.)
6. Refocus: Let's go back to this important message that Aki has begun to share – that disappointing you is very difficult for him, that he literally cannot hear you when he senses he has let you down.

Your Strengths and Discoveries about Catching a Bullet during Move 4 Processing

_____

_____

EFCT Tango Workout 7: Move 2 Assembly and Deepening Core Emotion in Stage 1

In this workout, you are given the opportunity to use Move 2 to help Aki discover, distil, and deepen the core fear driving his steps in the distress pattern with Mei-Ling.

Emily has validated Mei-Ling's disorientation at hearing Aki disclose that her shrill tone of voice listing his failures and her talk about feeling lonely triggers him to freeze with hearing she is disappointed in him, that he can no longer hear her words but that he simply goes numb. Now, she chooses to more deeply assemble Aki's fear of disappointing Mei-Ling. Emily is curious as you may also be, to more precisely understand what Aki is afraid of if Mei-Ling is disappointed in him.

AKI: I simply cannot hear her when her voice is loud. It is like my body is exploding with, "You've blown it. There is no chance. She is totally fed up with you," and my head freezes. I can't bear it and everything freezes! Or I tell her something rude and defensive like, "Ok this is a purely functional relationship where we each have our jobs to do and that's all." I go numb. When I'm numb I say, "I don't really care anymore."

Your Move 2 Assembly to Access Core Fear
  Link trigger, bodily response, action tendency, and meaning and then evoke the core fear by eliciting more about what it means when he says, "I can't bear it," in that split second just before everything freezes. (What can he not bear?): _____

_____

_____

Emily's Move 2 Assembly to Access Core Fear
  Mei-Ling's loud voice resounds through your entire body (trigger), your ears shut down and you go numb (body) and you want to get away from hearing how disappointed she is with you (action tendency/ meaning). Can you say more about that split second you simply cannot bear, before everything freezes and you go numb or say you just don't care anymore? Just before going numb what is happening?

Your Strengths and Discoveries about Move 2 Accessing and Distilling Core Fear

_____

_____

  Aki: (In response to Emily's evocative question, "Just before you go numb, what is happening?") I hear I've blown it. I have no chance. She has given up on me – rejected me. It's like I've already lost her. It's over! I'm under water with rocks on my chest.

Your Move 2 to Heightening his Core Fear

With RISSSSSC, repeat the trigger and use the emotional handle/kinesthetic image of *under water with rocks on my chest* to distill his attachment panic, and to deepen it._____

_____

_____

Emily's Move 2 Heightening Response

You hear Mei-Ling's loud voice (trigger) and you are immediately under water with rocks on your chest, drowning, flooded with a fear you've blown it, she's given up on you, and you've already lost her (core bodily felt attachment panic of her rejection). The fear of her rejection is just too much to bear. Underwater with rocks on your chest – no chance of survival without her. Your head and entire body freeze, even if you are saying you just don't care, inside you are frozen in panic that says she has given up on you and she is gone, do I hear you correctly?

Your Strengths and Discoveries about Move 2 Assembling, Distilling, and Heightening

_____

_____

EFCT Tango Workout 8: Move 3 to Shape an Engaged Encounter to Disclose Newly Accessed Core Emotion

In this workout, you are given the opportunity to SHAPE an encounter for Aki to disclose the core fear you helped him to discover, distil, and deepen with Move 2: His fear that Mei-Ling has totally rejected him/given up on him.

Insert your responses after each prompt, comparing with Emily's as you go. As before, you may wish to place a piece of paper over Emily's response, so you can make your own without interference.

Your Sharpening

Sharpen the core, assembled message to be shared with empathic tracking reflections of what was discovered, distilled, and deepened with Move 2: _____

_____

Emily's Sharpening

(Tracking reflections.) I want to help you share with Mei-Ling that underwater-rocks-on-mychest feeling that you have, when on the outside you may shrug or tell her this is just a functional relationship, but deep inside you are drowning with fear that she has rejected you and is giving up on you – and you have already lost her.

Your Heightening

Heighten the emotional experience of the message, repeating key elements of emotion, mirroring, and slightly heightening with RISSSSSC; using proxy voice also heightens present-moment experiencing: _____

Emily's Heightening
(RISSSSSC manner.) Under water, with rocks on my chest, hard to breathe, no idea how to keep you from giving up on me. Everything is a blur. I'll drown without you.

Your Anticipating
Using evocative responses and questions and repetition, help Aki to anticipate the experience of disclosing his fear to Mei-Ling and finding sufficient safety to do so: _____

_____

Emily's Anticipating
(To Aki.) Can you take a look at Mei-Ling just now. She has never seen this underwater fear. Can you imagine turning to her and telling her about this fear? (In proxy voice.) I may act as though I don't care, but hearing your loud voice telling me you feel alone and I have let you down – puts me under water with rocks on my chest. Disappointing you, letting you down, my entire body freezes with fear you are rejecting me.
(To Mei-Ling.) Mei-Ling, I know you haven't seen this side of Aki before. Can you listen to him tell you just now about drowning with fear on the inside when he may look on the outside like he doesn't care? (Mei-Ling is receptive and says she wants to hear from him.)

Your Directing to <u>Present</u>
Repeat the message and direct Aki to Present it to her: _____

_____

Emily's Directing to <u>Present</u>
(Focused direction to Aki.) Can you tell her, please, about drowning with fear that she is rejecting you, that you have let her down so much, she is giving up on you, how freezing and acting like you don't care is code for how frightening her loud complaints are for you – sending you drowning underwater with rocks on your chest?

Your Engaging
When Aki hesitates and says, "I can't imagine she's going to care about these rocks crushing me," re-engage him in his distilled experience, validating his fear that Mei-Ling will not care, and direct him again to share the message: _____

_____

Emily's Engaging
I hear how difficult it is to share with Mei-Ling that her words send you into this panicked place that she is disappointed with you. You can't imagine she will care to hear that your fear of disappointing her is like being underwater with rocks on your chest. She is having difficulty believing this new side of you, yes, but she has said she wants to hear from you, so can you take the risk please to let her see this side of you that truly cares about not letting her down?

Your Strengths and Discoveries about Move 3

_____

_____

EFCT Tango Workout 9: Move 4 Processing an Engaged Encounter

In Aki's engaged encounter to share his newly accessed core fear with Mei-Ling, his message and core fear expand and deepen while disclosing to her. When he tells Mei-Ling about his fear of disappointing her and experiencing her rejection, he adds:

> The worst of feeling crushed by these rocks while hearing your upset, is not only that I am drowning and hurting but that I have totally lost connection with you. Without you I am lost – without you, nothing matters anymore, and I am afraid you'd never want to help lift these crushing rocks.

After Aki's encounter with Mei-Ling, identify how you will savor the moment, checking with him how it was to share (repeating the core of what he shared) and then evoke Mei-Ling's internal experience as she received this disclosure from Aki. Experiment with repeating the core of the message Aki shared and any non-verbals you imagine from either partner each time you evoke their experiences.

Your Move 4 Processing with Aki _____

_____

_____

_____

Your Move Processing with Mei-Ling _____

_____

_____

_____

Emily's Move 4 Processing with Aki
You took this big risk to share with Mei-Ling, when you initially couldn't imagine she would care about these rocks crushing you. How was it to look right at her, with her looking back at you kindly and seemingly a little surprised and sharing your fears of disappointing her, and being rejected by her, and then with tears in your eyes to drop into your worst fear of all – that when you hear her raised voice and complaints of feeling alone, the heaviest crushing rock is your sense that you have totally lost connection with her and that without her you are lost? How was it to share that with her?

Emily's Move 4 Processing with Mei-Ling
You are looking rather shocked to hear all this from Aki. What is happening inside for you as you hear him describe that under his frozen face or what to you has so often looked like he didn't care, that he is feeling crushed and lost – having lost connection with you being his very worst fear – that without you he is lost? What comes up for you in your body, in your heart as you hear this from Aki?

Your Strengths and Discoveries about Move 4 Processing

_____

_____

Imagine Emily similarly does Tango Move 2 with Mei-Ling, to help her deepen her core underlying fear that drives her to become loud and aggressive (a word she herself used) toward Aki. Emily helps Mei-Ling assemble her core fear of being abandoned by Aki, being totally alone, and not at all precious to him.

Mei-Ling describes another trigger for her fear of being unloved by Aki: He will make love to her but he does not kiss her, and this sends her into a cascade of fear of being unlovable and unwanted. Then, envision that Emily, with Move 3, shapes an encounter for Mei-Ling to share this fear with Aki and, with Move 4, processes first with Mei-Ling and then with Aki who first expresses shock to see this frightened, vulnerable side of Mei-Ling and surprise to hear she wants his kisses. "You told me once you didn't like how I kissed you, so I have been playing it safe." He is pulled to respond with compassion and tenderness.

EFCT Tango Workout 10: Move 5 Integration and Validation

You have done workouts alongside Emily to lead Mei-Ling and Aki through the change event of de-escalation/stabilization and are preparing to move into Stage 2. How can you summarize the work they have done with a Tango Move 5, to validate and integrate the stabilization they have created? Insert your best attempt at a Move 5 summary to create coherence to their process this far. After doing so, compare with Emily's response, which may be different, but not better or worse than yours.

How to Do Move 5 Integration and Validation

- The goal of Move 5 is to integrate, validate, and summarize.
- It can be used in the midst of sessions and at the end of sessions.
- It can be used to summarize and heighten the corrective emotional experience of new moments of engaged contact.
- It often feels like a celebration, focusing on positive affect and emotional balance.
- During Stage 1, Move 5 is useful to draw the contrast between the old cycle or pattern and the new moves they are taking or even the ways they are now able to stop the old pattern and talk about what they are doing and the fears driving them.
- In Stage 2, Move 5 includes highlighting the new moves and emerging emotions, and emerging shifts in views of self and other, *broaden-and-build* patterns, and growing attachment security.
- In Stage 3, Move 5 summarizes, validates, heightens, and consolidates the impacts of the new resilience and secure bonds and the picture of the future on this trajectory.

Micro-interventions for Move 5 include empathic, tracking reflections of changes and change events, heightening, validating, and summarizing.

To create a Move 5 summary, contrast the escalation of the beginning of therapy with some of the new moves they have made so far. Include the coherence they are making of their action tendencies as code for underlying fears of abandonment or rejection; how they are each owning how they trigger one another and how they get triggered; the new views of each other that each one is beginning to see.

Your Move 5 Integration with Mei-Ling and Aki at this point in therapy _____

_____

_____

_____

_____

Emily's Move 5 Integration You have come a long way from where you began! You have each identified how you've gotten pulled off-balance into your repetitive push–pull pattern which used to leave you both frustrated and alone and feeling disconnected. Now, you Mei-Ling have been able to share with Aki that your loud, harsh, aggressive pushes are code for desperate attempts to get him to see you and respond to you, when underneath you are terrified you aren't precious to him any longer and you fear he is slipping away from you. Aki, you have been able to share with Mei-Ling, that you feel lost without connection with her and that happens each time she raises her voice. And you've shared that shrugging her off or walking away is code for your inner sense of drowning under crushing rocks of her disapproval and disappointment in you. You have new pictures of each other now. Mei-Ling you have a new picture of Aki as wanting to feel connected to you, and pulling away not because he doesn't care, but out of fear he cannot regain your approval. Aki, you have a new view of Mei-Ling, as wanting you, and becoming desperate and loud, not to reject you, but out of a panic to call you close. You both see that you value and want each other but become caught in creating and being hurt by this familiar, repetitive push–pull pattern.

Your Strengths and Discoveries about Move 5 _____

_____

_____

EFCT Tango Workout 11: Tango Move 1 to Enter Stage 2

How to Do Tango Move 1 to Guide A Stabilized Couple into Stage 2

1. Validate decreased reactivity and emotional balance, with tracking reflections of the present process. For example, "Now, when…" (name typical trigger), name how each is responding differently (action tendencies).
2. Identify the core emotions, fears, or longings that remain alive.

Read the couple's comments below out loud.

MEI-LING: Our weekends are going much more smoothly – at least when he is home and helping out with the kids. I don't feel alone all the time anymore, but… (pauses). I don't like getting loud and angry – but I still do. I still see that dazed look on his face sometimes – that tells me he is not hearing me and I get desperate to reach him and make him join in more! I start getting loud and louder, but then I stop and ask myself if I am overwhelming him again. Maybe he cannot hear me because I am sounding so aggressive… so I slow myself down and check in with him.

AKI: It is true, when she gets loud – when I hear I have let her down, again it's like my ears close up and I cannot hear – I just want to disappear or defend myself, and everything is a big blur… but I don't always do that anymore – I try very hard to listen to what she is saying, not to hear I'm the big let-down again.

Follow the prompts to form a Tango Move 1 to validate the emerging shifts and the lingering fears. After this, you can focus on Aki, the more withdrawn partner's core emotion to move into Stage 2.

Your Inner Process and Attunement

Identify the typical trigger for each partner:

Mei-Ling_____ Aki_____

Now, when the trigger happens, identify each one's different response, at least some of the time:

Mei-Ling_____ Aki_____

Identify the core emotions, fears, and longings still alive for each one:

Mei-Ling_____ Aki_____

Your Tango Move 1, reflecting present process at de-escalation, with emerging new views of self and other, new awareness of their part in their typical pattern, and emerging agency to interrupt the old pattern. Also, note the underlying fears that remain despite being less intense.

_____

_____

_____

_____

Emily's Inner Process and Attunement

Typical trigger for each partner: Mei-Ling's loud voice and complaints; Aki's dazed look

Different responses to trigger: Now Mei-Ling stops and asks herself if she is overwhelming Aki; now Aki keeps from disappearing or defending and tries to hear what Mei-Ling is saying

Core emotions, fears, and longings still alive: Mei-Ling remains afraid he is distancing/abandoning her; Aki remains fearful of disappointing Mei-Ling.

Emily's Move 1

Now when you see the dazed look on Aki's face that always told you he was not listening, you stop to check if you may be overwhelming him with your messages; now when Mei-Ling seems to be getting louder or is simply telling you how tired she is, you can listen to her without immediately getting overwhelmed and sensing you are disappointing her. Your ears don't close up so quickly anymore, and you can hear there is more to her words than disappointment or judgment of you. Even though your fears, Aki, of disappointing Mei-Ling and being rejected by her and your fears, Mei-Ling, of Aki disappearing and leaving you all alone, are still there, it sounds like your interactions are becoming much more satisfactory for both of you. You are not held hostage by that push–pull pattern all the time.

Your Strengths and Discoveries about Move 1 at De-escalation/Stabilization

_____

_____

EFCT Tango Workout 12: Move 2 Assembly and Deepening to Enter Stage 2

Aki and Mei-Ling have stabilized and de-escalated their problematic distress pattern. They are now moving into Stage 2 and your task in this Move 2 workout is to further assemble and deepen the core attachment fear of Aki, the more withdrawn partner. This fear, when it is most intense is his perception (meaning) that Mei-Ling doesn't love him or even like him and is about to reject him totally.

In Stage 1, he identified that this fear gets triggered when Mei-Ling raises her voice or expresses dissatisfaction or loneliness. His fear resurfaced as you did a Move 1, above, tracking the present de-escalated process and validating that his core fear remains.

Forming a Stage 2, Move 2 Assembly and Deepening Response
Your Inner Process and Attunement

Recall the coherence assembled in Stage 1 with Aki, that he does turn away or shrug his shoulders and do nothing when the sound of Mei-Ling's voice tells him she is disappointed in him. His ears shut down and he literally cannot hear her. He freezes with fear that she is rejecting him.

Resonate in your own body with Aki's internal experience of freezing in fear, going numb, terrified of rejection, and unable to breathe under the weight of the crushing rocks. How do you feel in your body as you resonate with this fear?_____

Your Stage 2, Move 2 Assembly and Deepening of Aki's Core Attachment Fear

1. With RISSSSSC, repeat an emotional handle. You can choose a bodily sensation he has described or another of his emotional handles. For example, "My ears shut down and I literally cannot hear her words;" "I am under water with rocks crushing me filled with terror she has already discarded me." _____

2. Evoke a felt sense of the fear that Aki acknowledges remains alive, with RISSSSSC (repetition, images, simple, soft, slow voice, somatic experience, client's words) and optionally, with an evocative question, evoke, expand, and deepen his present-moment experience:

_____

_____

Emily's Stage 2, Move 2 Assembly and Deepening of Aki's Core Attachment Fear

Option 1: What a dreadful fear to live within the background, even as you and Mei-Ling are starting to shift the old painful push–pull pattern! Her being upset with you is like rocks crushing on your chest, holding you underwater, terrified at any moment that the lady you love is giving up on you! Can you talk to me about how you feel that crushing fear in your chest just now? (Pause, giving him time to reflect inward.) And what does that pressure on your chest say in this moment?

Option 2: Those difficult moments when Mei-Ling's voice gets loud or expresses some dissatisfaction with you, your ears close down and as hard as you try, you cannot hear Mei-Ling's words above your panic that she giving up on you. You fear that nothing you do can win her favor again! Are you feeling that fear in this moment? (Pause) Where in your body? (Pause) And what does it say?

Your Strengths and Discoveries about Move 2 Deepening in Stage 2

_____

_____

EFCT Tango Workout 13: Move 3 in Stage 2 (Aki Taking Step 5)

Read Aki's words below aloud.

AKI: (Engaging more deeply with his core attachment panic.) This pressure says, "She doesn't even like me anymore." When I'm crushed under these rocks, I fear there is no hope for us. I don't trust she'd care to lift a rock crushing me, threatening to drown me – I think she'd be fine if the rocks simply crushed me til I couldn't breathe. I feel helpless. I can't even hear her words. I just freeze – can't bear it.

Now, SHAPE an encounter for him to share his newly deepened core emotion in a clear message to Mei-Ling. As before, consider covering Emily's responses until after you have inserted your own, unique response.

Your Sharpening
Use RISSSSSC to sharpen the expression of the core fear that was further distilled and deepened with Move 2: _____

_____

_____

Emily's Sharpening
(With RISSSSSC manner.) There are still these moments when Mei-Ling seems unhappy with you and the old fear gets triggered and, on the outside, you do nothing but shrug and walk away from Mei-Ling, but inside you are frozen with dread you have already lost her. I want to help you shape a message to tell Mei-Ling about this unbearable crushing terror that says she may not love you anymore; that your relationship is doomed and she has rejected you as a partner.

Your Heightening
Repeating key elements of emotion, heighten with RISSSSSC; using proxy voice also heightens preset-moment experiencing: _____

_____

_____

Emily's Heightening
(With RISSSSSC manner and proxy voice.) Any sign that Mei-Ling is disappointed with me, puts me underwater, rocks piled on my chest, hard to breathe, drowning without a sense of connection or love from Mei-Ling. Drowning with fear that she doesn't love me anymore – and I have already lost her, yes?

Your Anticipation
Using evocative responses and questions and repetition, help Aki to anticipate the experience of disclosing his fear to Mei-Ling and finding sufficient safety to do so: _____

_____

_____

_____

Emily's Anticipation
(With heightening and reflecting, to Aki.) Can you take a look at Mei-Ling just now? This crushing, underwater fear is deeper that she knows. Even though the two of you are doing so much better and you are showing up much more in the relationship, can you imagine turning to her and telling her about this fear, that you are working so hard to fight against? Can you let her know that when you sense you have let her down, this fear of losing her still puts you underwater with rocks on your chest and you simply cannot hear what she is saying?
(Turning to Mei-Ling.) Aki is experiencing this fear more deeply than before. Can you listen to him tell you just now about drowning with fear on the inside – this fear that you may not even love him anymore – that you might just let him drown under those rock? This fear that blocks his ears and he simply cannot hear you? Are you willing to hear this from him? (Imagine Mei-Ling is receptive and says she wants to hear from him.)

Your Direction to <u>Present</u> the Message
Repeat the message and direct Aki to Present it to Mei-Ling: _____

_____

_____

Emily's Direction to <u>Present</u> the Message
Can you see Mei-Ling's face – turning toward you? Can you tell her, please, about drowning with fear that she has stopped loving you and would let you drown crushed under rocks for letting her down so many, many times? This fear that gets so loud you cannot hear what her words are saying?

Your Engaging
Imagine Aki pauses to say, "I'm so sorry – I do try to hear you, but I cannot. I am drowning! I am sorry!" Refocus on his fear. Validate that, yes, he is very sorry, but re-engage and re-focus him on disclosing his newly deepened fear: _____

_____

_____

Emily's Engaging
You are sorry, yes. You want to hear Mei-Ling, and can you tell her that her messages of her disappointment in you are so strong that they deafen you, crush you and threaten to drown you? Can you share with her how lost and terrified you are that perhaps she has stopped loving you?

Your Strengths and Discoveries about Move 3 in the Beginning of Stage 2

_____

_____

_____

EFCT Tango Workout 14: Processing a Stage 2 Encounter with Move 4

Read Aki's engaged encounter with Mei-Ling aloud.

AKI: (Looking at Mei-Ling, with a stronger voice than when he was apologizing.) I am terrified of you giving up on me – (Short gasp to catch his breath.) that I've let you down too much…Afraid you see the rocks crushing me til I drown and you don't even want to lift a rock off of me. (Looking down.) It's heavy! (Takes another breath.) I hate that this fear deafens me, but (Pauses and voice raises ever-so-slightly.) but when I see, when I hear your discontent, I cannot hear you! I don't want to disappear from you!

Your Move 4 to Process This Encounter

Insert the key parts of Aki's disclosure and significant non-verbals that you choose to repeat, and invite him to describe his experience of sharing this with Mei-Ling:

_____

Next, insert your repetition of keywords and non-verbal parts of Aki's encounter again, and this time check with Mei-Ling about how she is experiencing Aki's disclosure to her:_____

_____

Emily's Move 4 Response to Aki

Your voice got stronger as you said to Mei-Ling, "I am terrified you have given up on me." How was it to tell her this and gasp for breath as you add that the rocks of fear crush you til you feel you will drown with no hope she'd care to lift a rock and to admit that when you hear her discontent, you simply do not hear her words? What is it like inside your gasping-for-breath body as you share this with her?

Emily's Move 4 Response to Mei-Ling

How was it for you, Mei-Ling, to listen to Aki, struggle to catch his breath as he shared this unbearably frightening experience of hearing your discontent with him? Hearing him tell you his fear that you'd let the rocks crush him til he drowns and to be so sorry that he simply cannot hear your words when he hears your discontent with him? That he does not want to disappear from you. What happens inside of you to receive this message?

Emily's notices Aki's hint of emerging assertiveness in his final words, where he paused and his voice raised ever-so-slightly as he said, "But when I see, when I hear your discontent, I cannot hear you!" It is important to notice this, because you will want to build on this assertive energy to facilitate his engagement and his request for her to tone it down so he can hear her.

His assertiveness will help to shift his view of other. When he experiences having a voice and being heard in a new way, his experience of her will begin to shift from her being unpredictable and dangerous, to becoming more predictable and trustworthy.

Your Strengths and Discoveries about Move 4 _____

_____

_____

EFCT Tango Workout 15: Move 3 to SHAPE the Unique Request Encounter *of the* Engagement Change Event (aka Step 7)

Aki has deepened and disclosed his core fear of rejection from Mei-Ling. In the previous workout, you processed this encounter, first with Aki and then with Mei-Ling. What would continue to be part of processing Mei-Ling's response to this deepened disclosure would be to help her integrate this emerging view of Aki as someone living in fear of letting her down, not wanting to disappear from her, and longing for her acceptance and approval. This is likely to continue to be challenging for Mei-Ling to take in and trust. In Workout 6, we practiced catching a bullet when she reacted with disorientation and mistrust to Aki's disclosure of this fear in Stage 1. She may continue to react with disbelief and disorientation, particularly to his emerging assertiveness. Helping Mei-Ling to integrate what Aki has shared, and validating her struggle if she is reactive, is part of her Step 6. Whether she is fully accepting of his emerging assertive, vulnerable disclosure or is struggling to trust it, the therapist will validate her experience, and shape an encounter for her to respond with an authentic encounter to share her experience. New views of one's partner are difficult to integrate. It is very risky to begin to trust what he is saying.

Then, it is time to shape another engaged encounter for Aki toward Mei-Ling. This encounter is to help Aki take the step of the engagement change event (Step 7) of stepping assertively into the relationship by making a request of Mei-Ling for what he needs from her to shift this fear that blocks him from fully participating in their relationship.

SHAPE (*sharpen, heighten, anticipate, present, engage*) the distinctive encounter of the engagement change event, where Aki asks Mei-Ling from an emotionally engaged place for what he needs to meet his attachment need. As suggested earlier, consider covering Emily's responses until after you have inserted your own.

Your Sharpening
Aki's attachment need is embedded in his fear. Repeat the fear and when he is clearly feeling the fear, evoke what the fear tells him he needs from Mei-Ling: _____

_____

_____

Emily's Sharpening
Let's tune into this paralyzing fear that arises with any sign that Mei-Ling is not happy with you and is rejecting you for letting her down. Let's listen to the fear that threatens to drown you and blocks you from hearing her and responding to her and see what this fear tells you that you need from Mei-Ling.

Your Heightening to Evoke the Need
Evoke and heighten Aki's need embedded in his core fear. Use RISSSSSC to keep the fear alive:

_____

_____

Emily's Heightening to Evoke the Need
Feeling crushed with fear of Mei-Ling rejecting you! When you are frozen and unable to respond to her or to even hear what she is saying, what do you need from her?

AKI: I need her to tone it down. Not get so angry with me when I slip up. Give me a chance to make mistakes. I do want to be with you. I want you to ease up on me so I can be safe to be myself with you.

Your Anticipation
Anticipate making the request. Using his words, help him prepare to ask her to ease up on him:

_____

_____

Emily's Anticipation
She is right there, listening to you. Right now, you have an opportunity to say, "I want to step in; I want to be safe with you…but I need you to ease up on me…give me some leeway to make mistakes."

Your Direction to <u>Present</u> the Message
Direct Aki to ask Mei-Ling for what he needs: _____

_____

Emily's Direction to <u>Present</u> the Message
Can you ask her? Can you ask her to ease up on you and give you a chance?

Your Engaging
Imagine Mei-Ling, interrupts, before Aki says anything, saying, "Of course I can do that." Refocus, to engage Aki. Give the directive again for Aki to ask Mei-Ling for what he needs:

_____

_____

Emily's Engaging
I'd like you to have the experience of asking her directly. And I'd like you, Mei-Ling, to experience Aki asking you for what he longs for from you. Can you, Aki, turn to her and ask if she is willing to ease up on you and give you a chance to make some mistakes?

Imagine Aki, makes this reach and requests of Mei-Ling, "Can you do this? Can you ease up on me and give me a chance to make mistakes? I want to be close to you. And I want to hear you and respond to you, but I need your acceptance. I am too weary of fearing your judgement and dreading your next tirade of discontent. Can you accept me and ease up on me? Tone down your voice?"

A Special Move 4 – To Invite Partner's Immediate Response

This calls for a special Move 4 after this unique *reach and request*. The therapist does not stop to process with the discloser and the receiver, but rather invites or allows the receiver to respond immediately to this request.

Emily, following Aki's clear request, prompts an immediate response from Mei-Ling: How do you respond to Aki's very clear request?

MEI-LING: I do want to accept you – I do. I want to ease up too – I hate my screeching tirades – I just need to know you are seeing me and hearing me. I don't want you drowning under a pile of crushing rocks. I want you to know I want you! I will try to tone down my voice and my criticisms.

After Mei-Ling's response to Aki's request, typical Tango Move 4 processing can follow, where the therapist processes Aki's experience of risking to reach, and checks if he can receive this tender response from Mei-Ling. Then, the therapist can process with Mei-Ling how it was to receive such a clear request from Ali of what he needs to come closer to her and remain engaged in the relationship. After processing with both partners, a Move 5 can be used to integrate, summarize, and celebrate this important change event of Engagement.

Your Strengths and Discoveries about Moves 3 and 4 to Shape the Step 7 Request

_____

_____

EFCT Tango Workout 16: Catching a Bullet with Move 4, During the Engagement Change Event

It is possible that Mei-Ling will melt with tenderness and compassion at Aki's disclosure as described above, however, it is common for this new level of vulnerability and assertiveness on the part of the engaging withdrawer to disorient a pursuing partner and for them to then respond with criticism. When disorientation or aggression arises, an EFT therapist *catches the bullet.* Imagine, the following, calling you to use the *catching bullet* type of conjecture. First, is a repeat of Aki's reach and request, followed by Mei-Ling's reactive response.

Read Aki and Mei-Ling's following words aloud to feel them in your body.

AKI: (Making this reach and request of Mei-Ling) Can you do this? Can you ease up on me and give me a chance to make mistakes? I want to be close to you. And I want to hear you and respond to you, but I need your acceptance. I am too weary of fearing your judgement and dreading your next tirade of discontent? Can you accept me and ease up on me? Tone down your voice?

MEI-LING: This seems over the top – I have never rejected you. Just asked you to be more present. I don't know if I can shower you with acceptance. What if you disappear again?

Your Attempt to Catch the Bullet
Validate Mei-Ling's disorientation while also heightening the assertive, engaged reach and request Aki has just made.

1. Interrupt Mei-Ling: _____
2. Reflect without judgment, in neutral, behavioral terms what just occurred: _____
3. Reframe the reactivity by conjecturing at confusion, disorientation, or disbelief_____

_____
4. Validate _____
5. Confirm with Mei-Ling: _____
6. Refocus _____

Emily's Attempt to Catch the Bullet

1. Interrupting Mei-Ling with validation: Of course this "new Aki" is hard to trust.

2. Reflecting in neutral, behavioral terms what just occurred: He just risked to you from the depths of his fear that you are giving up on him to let you know that he does want to be close to you, but that he needs your help – to tone down your voice and to give him reassurance and acceptance.

3. Reframing the reactivity by conjecturing at her disorientation, while restating the significance of his reach: You have never heard him show up with so much fear of losing you nor with such a clear request of how he needs your help to calm his fear of your rejection! So it must be quite disorienting to see this new side of Aki, yes?

4. Validating: Partly you feel blamed for doing something wrong and partly you are terrified that no matter what you do, he will disappear again, yes?

5. Confirm: Do I understand? (Pause for response. Mei-Ling nods, "Exactly!").

6. Refocus: Aki has just said to you that he wants to be close to you and that he needs you to give him a chance, to make mistakes; he is asking if you can ease up on him and tone your voice down. Can you respond to this request, please?

Your Strengths and Discoveries about Interrupting to Catch Bullets

_____

_____

Views of Self and Other

Imagine as was suggested above, that Mei-Ling made the reactive statement, "This seems over the top – I have never rejected you. Just asked you to be more present. I don't know if I can shower you with acceptance. What if you disappear again?" This brief statement carries implications of her negative view of self and other. It is important to make note of these views of self and other, because as you move toward facilitating her softening change event, they will reappear, and you will need to process them.

Insert what you notice about her implied view of self and other:
   View of other: _____; View of Self: _____

   What Emily notices: Emily hears implications of Mei-Ling's view of other as unreliable; cannot trust he will stay present and engaged; and of her view of self as a rejecting partner who asks too much and needs too much and is not capable of giving him what he needs.

EFCT Tango Workout 17: Move 5 to Integrate the Engagement Change Event

Imagine that after the therapist's support, whether or not there were bullets, that Mei-Ling does eventually respond with the response given at the end of Workout 15, and repeated here:

MEI-LING: I do want to accept you – I do. I want to ease up on you too – I hate my screeching tirades – I just need to know you are seeing me and hearing me. I don't want you drowning under a pile of crushing rocks. I want you to know I want you! I will try to tone down my voice and my criticisms.

In this workout, summarize, validate, integrate, and heighten or celebrate Aki's engagement change event, which incrementally emerged throughout their therapy, and was shown culminating in Workout 15.

Your Move 5 Response

Summarize what Aki and Mei-Ling have just done together. Feel free to use your imagination to add details to summarize. _____

_____

_____

_____

_____

Emily's Move 5 Response:

Amazing you guys! Aki, you spoke to Mei-Ling about the fear that crushes you and threatens to drown you – a terror that arises when you hear or see something from her that tells you she is unhappy with you! You shared your fear and she listened very intently. And then from within that fear, you found the clarity and the courage to ask her for what you need to soothe that fear so you can feel safer to engage openly with her. You asked her to ease up on you, to tone down what she calls her tirades and to assure you that she actually still loves you and likes you – that she can accept you as different from her.* And what a gift that was for you to hear Mei-Ling! You broke into a big, warm smile, with the kindest assurance that of course you accept Aki for who he is, that his reaching to you like this, makes you like him even more, but that you just need and want more of him! And Aki, you breathed a huge sigh of relief and said, "I really am starting to believe her."

* Option: In the event that Mei-Ling did not respond with such immediate warmth and there was a bullet to catch, Emily would say at that point: It was difficult for you, at first Mei-Ling. Your fears came up, wondering if he was painting you as a rejecting person – the one to blame here. And you also feared that even if you do help him he may disappear again. It was difficult to respond to him, but you did. You said, "I will try, I do want to try and tone my voice down so you can show up more with me." This is a new chapter for the two of you – Aki stepping in, telling Mei-Ling how you do want to be close to her, asking for her help and Mei-Ling, responding to this new openness from Aki, even as you are still afraid he could disappear!

Your Strengths and Discoveries about Move 5

_____

_____

_____

_____

EFCT Tango Workout 18: Move 2 with Mei-Ling, the More Pursuing Partner (Beginning Her Step 5)

Read Mei-Ling's following statement below aloud; resonate with her fear in views of other and self.

MEI-LING: He is much more present now. (Pauses.) Most of the time. (Smiles.) The kids are calmer, and we are happier! But I'm terrified this will not last. I am on the lookout for signs he's backing away. He just joined a new morning gym program and I'm not happy about that … What if he starts pulling away again? What if it's just an excuse to get away from me? (Pauses, looks down.) I can't trust he will stay close like this – so afraid this new Aki will not last…And arghh!! (Pauses) Yuck. (Pause.) I hate to say this, but, (twisting a tissue in her hands; voice cracking) I really am afraid I need him too much. Horrible. Pathetic really – who could want to stay close to someone this needy?

Your Inner Process and Attunement

First, identify your own personal reactions to Mei-Ling's expression. Then, identify Mei-Ling's trigger, bodily arousal, meanings, action tendencies, and core fears.

Your reactions: _____

Mei-Ling's elements of emotion: _____

Your Move 2 Assembly and Deepening. Recalling views of self and other that you identified at the end of workout 16, link elements of emotion into a coherent whole and deepen the core attachment fears in view of other and view of self:

_____

_____

_____

Emily's Inner Process and Attunement

Emily resonates with the positive newness emerging with Aki's more engaged presence. Emily has to admit to herself that her heart falls a little when she hears Mei-Ling, getting frightened by one more trigger. Then, she recalls this is typical for pursuers to be more fearful than ever as their partner engages. She attunes to how this is such a positive shift, while at the same time is of course raising many intense fears in Mei-Ling of "will he remain engaged" and "am I somehow defective?"

Emily's Move 2 Assembly and Deepening, especially of views of self and other:

You truly appreciate Aki being more present and closer to you (new cue) and at the same time, your voice breaks (bodily arousal) as you describe how frightened you are that this new closeness will not last (meaning/attachment fear). You are vigilant for little signs, "Is he really staying close to me or is he backing away?" (action tendency of checking for signs). His joining the new gym (cue) feels like an alarm bell, "Be careful – look out – what if he's pulling away – what if he is getting tired of being close to me," yes? (checking for confirmation while heightening her fear of abandonment/view of other being unreliable). You wring your fingers and blush and you put your deepest fear into words, "What if I am too much for him and he doesn't really want to be close to me?" (Again, a fear of abandonment, but this time negative view of self) (Deepening, with slow, soft tone, in proxy voice): "So afraid this amazingly present, new Aki will not last (view of other) and he'll pull away again, because I am too much (view of self)!"

Your Strengths and Discoveries about Move 2 in Stage 2 Assembly and Deepening

_____

_____

EFCT Tango Workout 19: Move 3 in Stage 2 (Helping Mei-Ling Continue Step 5)

Read Mei-Ling's following response aloud as if you were her, attending to the words and to the many non-verbal, somatic parts of her message.

MEI-LING: I am too much for him. I need too much! (Long pause!) How can he want to stay close to me? (Slow pace, voice breaking, tears streaming down her face). He will move away again ... always does ... I am too much! (Disgusted look on her face, wringing hands, placing hand on belly as though in pain.) I don't want him to see this pathetic side of me!

Now **SHAPE** (*sharpen, heighten, anticipate, present, engage*) an encounter for her to disclose her newly distilled and deepened core fears, related to view of self, view of other, and fear of reaching, in a clear message to Aki.

In this highly vulnerable encounter, *seeding attachment* is a very helpful micro-intervention. With seeding attachment, you heighten a sense of sufficient safety even as you heighten the fear. Your responses may be very different from Emily's and that is ok. The important thing is that you find a way to sharpen, heighten, anticipate, direct presentation of the vulnerable attachment fears, seeding attachment, slicing thinner, and re-engaging if/when needed.

Your Sharpening
Sharpen the fears Mei-Ling has to share with Aki, validating her present moment fear of being seen as unlovable and pathetic and of Aki moving away from her. Adding conjecture to your reflections may help to heighten and keep focus: _____
_____
_____

Emily's Sharpening
(Reflecting, validating, heightening, and conjecturing.) Let's see how we can shape this into a message to Aki, when letting him see you right now feels almost dangerous! So afraid to let him see how much you need him, yes? (Mei-Ling is twisting her fingers.) Your stomach churning with fear that he will move away again, like he did in the past. Disgust on your face, wondering if you are just too much for him to want to be close to you, yes?

Your Heightening
Using repetition and a slow, soft proxy voice, heighten the message to share: _____
_____
_____

Emily's Heightening
(Slow, soft, proxy voice.) So afraid he will take one look at me ... see me as pathetic because I need him too much... and he will be gone again! Don't show him. Don't let him see me like this. It's not safe!

Your Seeding Attachment to Anticipate
Use seeding attachment to help Mei-Ling anticipate the encounter. Heighten her fear with, "You can't imagine...," while also painting a picture of safety: _____
_____
_____

Emily's Seeding Attachment to Anticipate
You can't imagine sharing these fears with Aki, letting him see how very risky it is to let him see you just now, showing Aki how much you need him. You could never share these fears and ask him to come and soothe you? You can't imagine he would want to hold and comfort you when you feel pathetic, frightened, needy, yes?

Your direction to Present the Message
Direct Mei-Ling to present her core fears to Aki, slicing more thinly if needed: _____
_____
_____

Emily's direction to Present the Message
Can you peak at Aki just now, and can you see him tuning toward you right now? He is not pulling away. He is right here with you. Can you tell him how afraid you are that you need him too much – that he will take one look at you feeling this vulnerable and will disappear?

Scenario 1
Imagine that Mei-Ling says, "No, no, I cannot look at him. Too much. Too dangerous!" This calls for slicing it thinner. That is, to invite the client to share something that is less risky, but to say something that is totally congruent with their present-moment experience. Often this is, some form of, "Can you tell him, it is too difficult to share this with you right now?"
Your Engaging
Use slicing it thinner to engage Mei-Ling: _____
_____

Emily's Engaging
Too difficult to look at him now. Can you tell him, it is too difficult. I cannot tell you yet, how much I need you. I cannot tell you how afraid I am that I am too much for you.

Scenario 2
Emily invites Mei-Ling, "Can you peak at Aki just now, and can you see him tuning towards you right now? He is not pulling away. He is right here with you. Can you tell him how afraid you are that you need him too much – that he will take one look at you feeling this vulnerable and will disappear?" Imagine Mei-Ling looks up blankly and says, "I don't know what to tell him."
Your Engaging
Engage Mei-Ling when she goes silent and blank, use validation and slicing it thinner, to re-focus and engage her:_____
_____

Emily's Engaging
This feels like a life and death risk, so difficult to tell Aki how frightened you are that he will not like this tearful Mei-Ling who needs his comfort and care. He is right here listening. Can you tell him, please, "It's just too much right now to show you this fear."

Your Strengths and Discoveries about Move 3, to Help the Pursuing Partner Share Her Core Fear of View of Self, Fear of View of Other, and Fear of Reaching in Stage 2 _____
_____
_____

Following this, Mei-Ling shares a thin slice of her fear. Imagine more encounters follow, each with Move 4 processing. Mei-Ling shares her deepened core fear of abandonment from Aki (Step 5) and Aki is helped to process and respond to this vulnerability (his Step 6). It is time to shape yet another engaged encounter for Mei-Ling to make a vulnerable reach to Aki and request what she needs from him to transform this fear into felt safety and security.

EFCT Tango Workout 20: Move 3 to SHAPE the Unique Request Encounter of the Softening Change Event (Helping Mei-Ling Make the Step 7 Request)

This workout is to help the more pursuing partner, Mei-Ling, to make the vulnerable softening reach toward Aki to ask for what she needs to feel assured of the security of their bond.

Read Mei-Ling's words below; attune to the absolute panic in her last few sentences. Imagine how she looks as you read it aloud and resonate with what she must feel inside her body.

MEI-LING: (To Aki) Too difficult to let you see how much I need you. (Looks down.) It's like removing all my protection, like stepping out of my skin and letting you see how ugly I am. Terrified you'll just walk away. Reaching to you when I need you this much is foolish (Pauses, wraps her arms around her body). My skin is burning! I will die!

Now, using EFT micro-skills SHAPE an encounter for Mei-Ling to make a request for Aki to meet the need embedded in her fears. *Seeding attachment* is very helpful to keep the fears of view of self, view of other and of reaching alive, while also seeding hope and possibilities of secure bonding.

SHAPE the unique encounter of the softening change event:

Your Sharpening
Sharpen the search for Mei-Ling's attachment need embedded in her fear. Repeat the fear and make an evocative response: _____

_____

_____

Emily's Sharpening
Reaching to Aki when your skin is burning with fear of how much you need him seems foolish. Reaching to ask him to be with you when you need him this much feels like suicide. You will be totally exposed, without any protection, without skin, and you see him turning away. You can't imagine he'd like to see you so raw, so vulnerable, and want to come a protect you? So difficult to imagine he would stick right by you? Too hard to reach to ask him to stay with you and protect you, yes? (Seeding attachment.)

Your Heightening to Evoke the Need
Evoke and heighten Mei-Ling's need embedded in her core fear: _____

_____

_____

Emily's Heightening to Evoke the Need
When your skin burns with terror that you are unsafe alone… When you are so uncertain Aki can love you the way you are just now, what do you need from him?

Imagine Mei-Ling says, "I need him to come and be with me; hold me and stay with me to keep me safe!"

Your Anticipating
Help Mei-Ling to imagine asking Aki for what she needs: _____

_____

_____

Emily's Anticipating
So vulnerable and alone, feeling all, you need is for Aki to come and hold you and tell you he will stay with you. Can you picture that if you asked him and he came, to hold you, you would be safe?

Your Direction to Present the Request Encounter
With encouragement and persistence, invite Mei-Ling to ask Aki for what she needs: _____

_____

_____

Emily's Direction to Present the Request Encounter
Can you ask him, please? Can you see he is leaning in – right here with you – Can you ask him to come and hold you and assure you he will stay with you because he wants to be with you?

Imagine Mei-Ling hesitates, and Aki comes to the rescue and says, "Of course I can do that. It is all I have ever wanted is to know she needs me!"

Your Engaging
Slow down, respectfully validate the process, and refocus, giving the directive for the encounter again: _____

_____

_____

Emily's Engaging
It is risky to ask, and Aki is right here responding before you even ask, but I'd like you to experience taking the risk – like jumping off a cliff and finding out how good it is to have Aki catch you and reassure you that you are the one he wants and he is there to catch you if you jump. Can you do it? Can you ask him directly to come and be with you? To hold you and to stay with you to keep you safe? Can you ask him to assure you he loves you in all your weaknesses and tears and that he will not be scared away anymore?

Your Strengths and Discoveries about Move 3 to Help the Pursuing Partner Make this Pivotal Reach _____

_____

_____

Following this unique encounter, imagine a special Move 4 where Aki makes an immediate response of assurance to Mei-Ling's reach/request. This is also discussed at the end of Workout 15, following Aki's request to Mei-Ling.

Then, the typical Move 4 would be used to process Mei-Ling's experience in having taken this enormous risk with Aki, one she could barely take because the stakes were so high, and to be met with Aki's more-than-eager reassurance and quick move to hold her and protect her. Aki's experience of this encounter will also be processed.

Move 5 would be used to summarize, validate, and heighten this watershed third change event of EFT. The Softening change event will be integrated and the new secure bond between Aki and Mei-Ling will be consolidated in Stage 3 as their newly secure bond and *broaden-and-build* pattern is integrated across pragmatic issues in their lives.

Having reached the final EFCT Tango workout, you can be assured your EFT muscles have been toned and strengthened. When you encounter a quandary in your EFCT practice, or a couple appears blocked, refer to the *list of EFCT Tango Workouts on p. xi*. Watch your video or read your notes to locate where your couple is on the map of EFT change. Insert their words and non-verbal communication into the relevant workout and let it guide you to workout with these EFT micro-skills and moves in the EFT Tango.

PART 2.3: EFIT TANGO WORKOUTS WITH SAMIR

In the introduction to Part 2 of this book, the five moves of the EFT Tango are described in detail and EFIT examples of each move with an individual named Keiko are given. You may want to reread that introduction (Part 2.1) as a refresher of the five moves before beginning the EFIT Tango Move workouts below.

This series of EFIT Workouts provides you with opportunities to apply all the EFT micro-interventions in the EFT Tango with Samir, a Palestinian immigrant who moved from a refugee camp in Hebron, with his parents, to Canada, at the age of two. He and his wife had been best friends since elementary school and it was always their dream to return to Palestine for several months to a year for their daughters to have an Arabic immersion experience and to experience life in a Palestinian refugee camp, to truly know their roots and to integrate Arabian values.

Flowing with moves of the EFT Tango, you will work with Samir through 22 workouts. Beginning with identifying goals and longings to find focus, the workouts extend from the beginning of therapy through Stages 1 and 2, ending with an opportunity to form a Move 5 to summarize and validate his corrective emotional experiences, which culminate in restructuring his working models of self and other and shape a new broaden and build pattern of emotion regulation.

EFIT Tango Workout 1: Identify Client Goals and Longings to Find Focus

To prepare for attuning and engaging with Samir with the EFT Tango Moves, please read the paragraph below and Samir's words to identify the goals and longings you hear Samir to be conveying.

When he enters therapy, Samir is a single parent of two teenage daughters and is suffering from a chronically depressed mood, lack of motivation, and little sense of meaning in life. He works as a journalist, and perceives he is passed over for jobs for which he has many strengths. He begins therapy saying he is tedious of diagnostic labels that keep him spinning in a sense of being abnormal; he feels stuck in a rut. He wants to make changes – to feel more confident, have more of a sense of purpose in life, and enjoy his teenage daughters' enthusiasm and joy for life. A few of the labels that he feels weigh him down are *chronic depression, complex PTSD, narcissistic abuse survivor*, with the latter referring to his experiences with his father, and *prolonged grief disorder* with regard to the death of his wife, five years earlier.

SAMIR: Of course, I am in grief, but we are moving on. And, yes, my father was difficult, but I know he suffered a lot growing up in a refugee camp and working for the Red Crescent Society, but I just have to move on. I definitely want to be a better father than he was and I believe I am. Not really interested in labeling him a narcissist or me a survivor of narcissistic abuse or a victim of prolonged grief. I don't want to search for what is wrong with me. I want to move forward. I must rebuild my life from this rubble and find some meaning again!

Your Identification of Goals and Longings Samir Is Conveying
Insert the longings and goals you hear and that you will use to focus your work with Samir. Phrase them positively and tangibly – as concrete, visible, tangible, realistic goals, and not simply what he wants to get away from or have less of. For example, "to enjoy his daughter's laughter" is a positive, concrete, tangible goal. "To be less depressed" or "to stop shutting out his daughters" are goals that are negative (the absence of something), intangible, and cannot be visualized.

_____

_____

After inserting the goals you hear, compare with what Emily hears, below. Yours may be different and that is ok. What matters is that you hear one or two goals in the client's story that can give you a focus for your work ahead.
Emily's Identification of Goals and Longings

Emily hears a longing from Samir to move from a sense of spinning in "what is wrong with me" to getting focused on a path forward out of the rubble of depression into a world where he feels confident, has a sense of purpose, can enjoy his daughters' enthusiasm and zest for life, and is free from the oppressive effects of his grief. She also hears two longings that may be too far on the leading edge for Samir at this point: to explore and find peace with the formative relationship with his father and to discover an alive connection with his now-deceased wife.

Your Strengths and Discoveries Identify what you liked about the goals you chose and anything you'd like to integrate from what Emily did: _____

_____

_____

Each workout with Samir ends with space for you to identify your "strengths and discoveries" – what you liked about the intervention you formed and what you discovered from Emily's response that you may want to integrate into your style.

EFIT Tango Workout 2: Move 1, Reflecting Present Process

Reflecting the Pattern (Triggers and Action Tendencies) and Hints of Disregarded Core Emotion in This Pattern

Directions for doing each move are provided the first time that move is introduced. After that, only prompts are given.

How to Do Move 1 Reflecting Present Process

1. Attune to the pattern of *trigger and action tendency* and to the emotional impact of this pattern.
2. Resonate – in your own body with:
   a. the triggering experience (likely the actions of others or other contextual events) and
   b. how the client responds (action tendency).
   c. If you have not yet identified the trigger and the action tendency, continue to be curious to discover both the trigger the client perceives as threatening or challenging and the client's action tendency. Pure empathy for how difficult a situation may be for a client without understanding *what triggers them and how they are responding to the threatening cue is not enough. We are collaborating with clients to identify their <u>strategies/patterns</u>. It is empowering for clients to explore the patterns of how they are engaging with life – with self, with others, and with the context of their experience.*
3. Find words and use the client's words to formulate the link between trigger and action impulse. "The more... the more..."
4. Check for confirmation that your words match the client's experience. Verbally ("Yes?") or non-verbally (with tentativeness through voice inflection) invite the client to confirm, adjust or correct your words (communicated empathic understanding).

Most workouts contain: (1) An expression from Samir; (2) prompts for you to insert your inner process and attunement; (3) space to insert your tango move; (4) samples of Emily's inner process and attunement; (5) Emily's EFT Tango move; (6) space to insert your strengths and discoveries when you compare your responses to Emily's. A further response from Samir sometimes follows.

Read Samir's comments below aloud as though you were him. Then, follow the directions to form a Tango Move 1 response. An EFT therapist is likely to intersperse reflections into this story as the client tells it, but to give you a sense of Samir's experience, you can read all of this out loud without any therapeutic reflections.

SAMIR: I feel I'm a disappointment at work. Ever since I turned down the assignment in the Middle East, I don't feel a part of things anymore; I can't say what I'd like to say to my colleagues...especially to my boss. I go silent and then I get grumpy. I don't even share my good ideas anymore – not sure I actually have many... (Voice trails off, then he continues.) I used to enjoy chatting with my boss. We came up with a lot of creative ideas, but he was disappointed with me when I said no to the Middle East assignment... (Pause.) ... so everything has changed. (Brief sigh.) I have nothing to say... no ideas.... getting hard to parent too – too hard. But what can you do? (Shrugs his shoulders.) It is what it is! I get impatient with my daughter at times – they are terrific, but sometimes I lose my patience and start to yell – I hate that. (Hangs his head.) I see their excitement, hear their laughter but I can't join in. I'm very tired and lonely. Their mother was killed when we were in Palestine. (Long pause.) I blame myself some days… But that was a long time ago! Five years, actually. (Longer pause, wipes a tear.)…. I feel like a wounded animal… too afraid to let anyone close, so it keeps running away or scaring others off.

Your Inner Process and Attunement

1. Most poignant emotional impact communicated: _____
2. Identify what triggers and threatens Samir: _____
3. Identify what Samir does in response: _____
4. Your bodily resonance with this pattern: _____

Your Tango Move 1. Use behavioral, nonjudgmental words. You may indicate where you would pause in your response, to check if your words are accurately capturing Samir's experience. Formulate the link between trigger and response (optionally adding emotional impact of the pattern):

_____

_____

For this workout and each of the following workouts, create your Tango Move; read it aloud; read Emily's inner processes; read her EFT Tango response aloud. Compare your responses to discover your strengths and new aspects you want to add to your style.

Emily's Inner Process/Attunement

1. The most poignant emotional impacts that Emily attunes to with Samir are his loneliness, his grief, and the brief tear and emotional experience he wipes away, all captured in the poignant image of his emotional pain: *A wounded animal, hurting but afraid to let anyone close, running away or scaring others off.*
2. Emily identifies triggers and responses unfolding before her:
   <u>What triggers/threatens Samir:</u> something happens at work in the way his boss or colleagues act around him; his daughters' excitement and laughter; the tragic loss of his wife, five years ago, that he blames himself for; facing life as single parent
   <u>What Samir does in response (action tendency):</u> isolates, dismisses his own pain, gets inpatient with his daughters, blames himself
   <u>Emily's resonance with this pattern:</u> She feels an emptiness in her own stomach as she sees Samir feeling loss and loneliness, feeling like a wounded animal, at work and at home, needing care, yet mistrusting letting others close to him; barely trusting to feel his grief and wondering if he is to blame.

Emily's Tango Move 1 Emily wants to avoid words that may convey judgment. She also wants to stay very close to his experience and avoid conjecturing beyond what he has offered.
   Example 1 (Focused on the pattern–triggers and the active process of numbing.)
   Sounds like you shut down a lot – the more you notice something about how your boss or colleagues relate to you, or you hear your daughters' laughter, the more you shut down, or move

away from others and from yourself. (Pauses to check for Samir's response to indicate of he is feeling understood.) "It is what it is," you say, and shrug your shoulders. The numbness takes over quickly, yes? And like a wounded animal, you don't let anyone close and you begin to wonder if you are scaring others away or if are you running away from them. Is that how it goes?

Example 2 (Focused on the loss and pain at the edges of his pattern of isolating from others and his own pain.)

Such a prison of loss and loneliness you feel caught in. Feeling so much pain over the loss of your wife and your losses at work since you turned down the Middle East travel. The more alone you are as a single parent and distant from colleagues at work, the more you isolate, feeling left out, unable to join in the laughter with your daughters, brushing away your own tears at missing your wife (She pauses to make sure Samir feels she is accurately reflecting his emotional process and experience).

You feel the wounds of your losses, knowing you need others' help, yet you find you keep at a safe distance from others, and from your own pain as well, yes? Sounds like a vicious cycle: The more you isolate, the less others come to you, the less others come to you, the more you mistrust and isolate. Am I getting it?

Your Strengths and Discoveries about Move 1

_____

_____

SAMIR: Exactly – I'm caught in this cruel spin.

Emily takes note of Samir's description of the pattern that is currently holding him prisoner – another emotional handle (a cruel spin). She simply repeats it, with a tone of heightening: A very cruel spin, indeed!

EFIT Tango Workout 3: Move 2 Assembling Emotion in the Pattern with Tracking Reflections

How to Do Move 2 Assembly

Tracking explicit elements of emotion, expanding elements, and evoking hidden elements of emotion:

1. Identify *an emotional/cultural handle* that strikes you as the salient part of the message, to expand.
2. Repeat it aloud and get the feel of this *emotional handle* in your own body.
3. Notice the explicit elements of emotion the client is conveying; consider:
   a. What is the cue/trigger that signals a threat?
   b. What are the somatic reactions (facial or bodily movements)?
   c. What is the client saying about meanings they are making?
   d. What are the client's action tendencies?

e. What elements are missing or are very general and you will want to evoke, expand, or deepen?

4. Repeat the elements in a vivid, specific manner, matching the client's emotional tone. Then, make a clear invitation to expand on a specific hidden element or to invite more specific exploration of a vaguely stated element (such as: Tell me more about…).

Read Samir's comments below aloud. To give you a sense of Samir's experience, you can read all of this out loud without any of the therapeutic reflections which would be likely in real life.

SAMIR: I am caught in a cruel spin feeling unpredictable most days, swinging from my cold, lonely, dark isolation where it is quiet and safe, to having random rageful outbursts! Outbursts at my daughters and on occasion, even at work. I want a meaningful life but mostly I live in numbness and in a dark cloud of depression that comes for me. At work, I feel marginalized. I'm convinced I am passed over for jobs I would be good at – but ever since I turned down that assignment in the Middle East, I may as well be invisible! My skin tone doesn't help either, I am sure (pause) I never quite belong. My boss gives me the cold shoulder and people carry on as though I am not there.

Because I speak French, English, and Arabic, I was the perfect person for that assignment, but I couldn't leave my daughters; they were too young for me to leave them. They are my life! (He beams briefly as he refers to them). I concede now. I fold into myself. Basically, don't say much. (Body slumps ever-so-slightly.) I have no impact or respect in my office anymore. Mostly I push it aside – nothing I can do, try not to be bitter, but I guess I really am bitter! I do have something to offer in that office – if only they would listen to me! (back stiffens, sits straighter, volume increases). I had good reason to turn down the job because I put my daughters first!

Your Inner Process and Attunement for a Move 2 Assembly

1. Identify the explicit elements of Samir's emotional experience he has expressed. Beside each element you identify, indicate what additional specificity needs to be evoked, with Move 2 evocative responses or questions.

Examples:
Perceived threatening cue: <u>Boss' cold shoulder</u>; **Evoke**: <u>What does his boss do that feels like a cold shoulder?</u>
Meaning made: <u>I have no impact</u>. **Evoke**: <u>What do others do that tells you that you have no impact?</u>

Threatening cue: _____	Expand or evoke?	_____
Bodily reaction: _____	Expand or evoke?	_____
Meaning made: _____	Expand or evoke?	_____
Action tendency: _____	Expand or evoke?	_____

2. Identify any hint of attachment panic or core, unexpressed emotion that you hear:

_____

Your Move 2 Assembly
   Link these elements together in a Move 2 tracking reflection: _____

_____

_____

Emily's Inner Process and Attunement for a Move 2 Assembly

1. Emily attunes to elements of emotion Samir has already identified:

Perceived threatening cues/triggers: Boss gives him the cold shoulder (Emily notes that she is not clear what this looks like, so she will want to evoke more about what actually happens that he perceives as a "cold shoulder"); Has no impact in the office (Emily notes she is also unclear how that looks in practice). Emily wants to evoke more specifics, about what his boss, and others in office do, which conveys to Samir he is invisible and has no impact.
Body: Hangs his head when speaks about losing his temper at work and with his daughters; slumps in his chair when talking about conceding and having no voice, no impact at the office; straightens his back when he says, "I do have something to offer!" and, "I had good reason – put my daughters first!" (Emily wants to expand on this spark of confidence.)
Meaning: I'm ignored, passed over, have no value, no impact; I had good reason to turn down the assignment because I needed to put my daughters first! He discovers as he acknowledges his bitterness that there is a spark of confidence he has been ignoring, "I do have something to offer!" (Emily hears his bitterness and confidence and wants to expand on it.)
Action tendency: Folds in on himself, concedes and does not speak up for himself; occasionally loses his temper; acknowledges he is bitter; expresses a spark of confidence he has been ignoring. (Emily hopes to expand Samir's ownership of these action tendencies.)

2. Emily hears hints of Samir's attachment panic (more meaning): Feeling invisible, de-valued, rejected; bitterness implies some anger or a voice that wants to be heard but fears no one will listen. In that core anger is a hint of confidence or assertiveness.

Emily's Move 2 Assembly
   Emily's tracking reflection to assemble these elements into a coherent story, before evoking more specifics: You experience your boss as giving you the cold shoulder (cue) and that you have no impact in your office. This says to you that you are invisible, ignored (meaning) You drop your head when you speak of losing your temper (body), yet your spine straightens (body) when you say, "I do have something to offer! I had good reason to put my daughters first!" Mostly you fold in on yourself and do not speak up but in your voice and in your body is a spark of confidence that you still have much to offer. Am I following you correctly?

Your Strengths and Discoveries about Move 2 Assembly

_____

_____

EFIT Tango Workout 4: Evoking More Specificity in Move 2 Assembly

In Workout 3, you identified elements of emotion about which you want to expand and evoke more specificity. Insert some evocative questions or responses you could use for this purpose:

_____

_____

Now read Emily's Move 2 evocative responses below as she helps Samir expand and makes his emotional experience more explicit and alive.

EMILY: (To elicit more about the triggers for Samir's perceptions of rejection at the office) *Can you tell me more about what your boss and your colleagues do that looks cold, distant, and* devaluing?

SAMIR: They don't discuss exciting projects anymore. I'll get an email about a new assignment but it's all factual – directives – still plenty of work for me – but since I don't want to travel far, they seem disappointed in me. I've even overheard someone say, "Samir would have been the perfect guy for that job, but…" and then their voices quiet down. Being a single parent certainly has its stigma. Or it is my skin tone? I'm ignored, left out (brief look of sadness crosses his face).

EMILY: (To evoke more about this present-moment sense as his body straightens and his voice increases in volume) Did you notice your body straighten and your voice become louder (bodily signs of emerging emotion) as you said, "I couldn't leave my daughters. I guess I am bitter. I do have something to offer!" And tell me more about the bitter experiences of being ignored and left out because of your skin tone.

SAMIR: I hadn't noticed – but yes, there is a spark of confidence in my bitterness. It's like I want to shout, "Listen to me!" Whether they are excluding me because of the stigma of my parenting responsibilities or because of my color, I am confident I still have much to offer and I do not like to be ignored!

Continue Move 2 Assembly (linking elements of Samir's emotion together with his newly emerging core emotion of anger/bitterness): _____

_____

_____

_____

_____

Emily's Continuing Move 2 Assembly

Linking these elements, Emily continues: Sadness crosses your face as you speak of the exclusion you experience, wondering, "Is it my skin color or my being a single parent that leaves me on the outside?" and then your voice gets louder and stronger as you exclaim, "Seems no one recalls how much I have to offer!"

Your boss and your colleagues carry on without checking in with you. They seem cold and distant (trigger) and your immediate reaction is to concede, get quiet, and fold in on yourself (action tendency, body). You tell yourself no one at work values you; no one even sees you (hint of attachment panic). You fear (more meaning) that this cold treatment is because you turned down the job in the Middle East, but when you say, "I couldn't leave my daughters?" your energy comes alive. It is like you are saying, "I am bitter! I had good reason to turn down the job because I put my daughters first!" It's like you discover a spark of confidence that you have been ignoring, and you say, "I do have something to offer! I want them to notice me and hear me!" yes?

Your Strengths and Discoveries about Move 2

_____

_____

SAMIR: (Smiles) Yes, I have been so afraid they were fed up with me (rubs his hands on his heart) – that they didn't like that I said no to the Middle East travel assignment and I've felt terrible and unworthy. I was disappointed too that I couldn't accept that assignment but when I hear you say that I don't speak up at work but that I am certain I did the right thing, that is so true! My daughters are important to me! I feel it every day but I try to ignore it, because then I begin to think of how much I miss my wife and I can't go there! (Shifts in his chair.) And I know I made the right decision about not taking the Middle East assignment – but it's too much –too much – just need to carry on.

Emily has been wondering if she is moving toward shaping an encounter with his daughters or with his boss or a colleague because work and parenting seemed like two equally important relationship contexts, when suddenly Samir introduces another relational context with "*how much I miss my wife and I can't go there.*" She recognizes she needs to take time to briefly acknowledge the new emotional handle of the relationship context Samir has introduced. She wants to be clear they will return to it and to be transparent about staying with the process they are presently assembling. Before *deepening* in Workout 6, we interrupt the process to (1) identify Samir's relational contexts of which we are aware and (2) be transparent about the process.

EFIT Tango Workout 5: To Identify Different Relational Contexts

You have two workout tasks in Workout 5: Identify different relational contexts in which Samir's repetitive protective pattern recurs; be transparent with him about the therapeutic process.

Your Inner Process and Attunement to Samir's Relationship Contexts

What relationship contexts are presently apparent for Samir, in addition to his work-context, that you can identify? Picture Samir holding different relationship balloons with a similar emotion regulation pattern of pushing aside his troubling thoughts and emotions. In what other relationships do you anticipate you may be exploring his emotion regulation pattern of getting triggered and avoiding? This is not to share with him, but rather to fine-tune your awareness of the different relational contexts in which his pattern of avoidance is active.

_____

_____

_____

_____

Emily's Inner Process and Attunement to Identify Samir's Relationship Contexts

Emily makes a note of multiple *relationship balloons* to explore, in which Samir is likely to have a similar emotion regulation pattern of getting triggered by others and reacting by holding back and muting his own voice. While she expects more key relationship stories are likely to emerge in their work together, the relationships she is aware of thus far include: work relationships; Samir's relationship with his daughters and the pattern with them; the grief/relationship with his deceased wife and the pattern in his relationship with her; his internal relationship with his own emotions of grief and loss; his brief reference to his harsh father whom he does not want to blame; finally, there is his ongoing relationship with Emily, his therapist.

Your Strengths and Discoveries about Identifying Different Relational Contexts

_____

_____

Your Transparency about the Process

How could you be transparent with Samir about your therapeutic intentions/process while acknowledging you have heard his poignant emotional handle of "how much I miss my wife – and I can't go there" and return to completing Move 2 assembly and deepening the core emerging emotion in the emotion you have assembled with him?

_____

_____

_____

Emily's Transparency about the Process

To continue to create safety and foster the task alliance with Samir, while doing more Move 2 assembly and deepening, Emily is transparent that she heard this poignant emotional handle of "how much I miss my wife but I can't go there":

It seems like this is the way you've learned to deal with the difficult things that you've survived: - pushing away difficult thoughts and feelings when they arise. And your wife's loss seems particularly unbearable. I hear how much you miss your wife and it feels just too much right now – I hear you are not ready yet to explore that deep loss. We will come back to that when you are ready. (Seeding attachment, picturing, by implication, a hope that eventually he will be ready to explore his deep loss of Nahlah). For now, I'd like to stay with the new certainty I hear emerging from the fear that you are being judged for having declined the Middle East assignment. As your body shifts in your chair, you say clearly, "I know I made the right decision about not taking that Middle East assignment!"

Your Strengths and Discoveries about Being Transparent about the Therapy Process

_____

_____

EFIT Tango Workout 6: Move 2 to Deepen Awareness of Samir's Emotion Regulation Pattern and His Emerging Core Emotion

> ### How to Do Move 2 to Deepen Emotional Engagement
>
> 1. Identify an *emotional handle* that captures the *emotion-story* assembled thus far. The emotional handle can be bodily movements, images, or poignant phrases.
> 2. Resonate with how this emotional handle feels in your own body.
> 3. Slowly and simply repeat the assembled *emotion-story*, optionally in proxy voice. Resist inferences and conjectures. Matching the client's emotional tone is likely to evoke a slightly deeper level than what the client has conveyed.
>
> This newly coherent, deepened, simplified whole, is likely to prime the client for an encounter.

Prepare to deepen Samir's pattern of emotion regulation and his hint of newly emerging core, assertive anger as it plays out in his context of exclusion at work. His pattern is what he calls the "cruel spin" of "the more he experiences others excluding him, the more he goes quiet and folds in on himself, fearing judgment and unworthiness, and the more others distance, and on and on." This pattern of going quiet and "folding in upon himself" ironically protects him from his core fear of rejection and of being a disappointment; it also protects him from experiencing his core assertive anger that could make him vulnerable to more rejection in his work context.

Below are Samir's words again that you read earlier, before the therapist transparency of promising to return to how much he misses his wife, when he is ready to do so. Read them aloud.

SAMIR: I am so afraid they are fed up with me (rubs his hands on his heart), that they didn't like that I said no to the Middle East travel assignment. I feel terrible and unworthy and just go silent. I am disappointed too that I couldn't accept that assignment! But when I hear you say I don't speak up at work but that I am certain I did the right thing, that is so true! My daughters are important to me! I feel it every day – but I try to ignore it, because then I begin to think of how much I miss my wife – and I can't go there! Shifts in his chair – And I know I made the right decision about not taking the Middle East assignment – but it's too much – wanting to be a good parent and wanting to shine at work! ARGH!! It's a jumble – too much. I just need to carry on.

Your Inner Process and Attunement, for Move 2 Deepening

1. Identify an emotional handle: _____
2. Identify Samir's bodily signals: _____
3. Resist inferences and conjectures.
4. Identify your bodily resonance: _____

Your Tango Move 2 to Deepen Awareness of His Emotion Regulation Pattern and Emerging Core Emotion

Heighten the *assembled emotion-story* of Samir's pattern, linked to his core emotion. After inserting it, read it aloud. _____

_____

Emily's Inner Process and Attunement, for Move 2 Deepening:

1. Emotional handle: "I know I made the right decision, choosing to stay with my daughters!"
2. Emily notes that Samir's body shifts and his voice becomes louder.
3. Emily resists conjecturing and inferring beyond Samir's expressed fears of rejection and the core assertive anger and confidence he has expressed. She wants to engage with and deepen the core emotions he has already expressed.
4. Emily's felt sense is one of solidness/strength amidst Samir's fears of rejection, loneliness, and experienced exclusion, and at the same time, she senses it is frightening to express confidence or anger.

Emily's Move 2 to Deepen Awareness of His Emotion Regulation Pattern and Emerging Core Anger/Assertiveness. (Speaking in proxy voice, to his boss.)

So afraid you are disappointed with me – that I have let you down. Afraid too of letting you down more, so I lie low and start to doubt myself. But I'm getting so tired and lonely in my hideout, knowing I still have a lot to offer! (Out of proxy voice): Samir, you speak of this cruel spin of your self-protective pattern – lying low and doubting yourself, and yet, beneath the pain of exclusion is this feisty confidence that feels deep within that you did make the right decision and you do still have a lot to offer, yes?

Your Strengths and Discoveries about Move 2 Deepening _____

_____

_____

Can you sense how this process of creating coherence and deepening of the *emotion-story* can help clients make nonjudgmental sense of their action tendency, in context, and prime them for an engaged encounter?

EFIT Tango Workout 7: Move 3 Shaping an Engaged Encounter to Own Action Tendency and Core Emotion

SHAPE a Move 3 Encounter for Samir to own his action tendency to lie low and pull away from others, in the context of his fears of being a disappointment, being unworthy, unwanted perhaps, he concludes, because of the tone of his skin or because of how he puts his parenting responsibilities ahead of job advancement, or both, but with a growing irritation that hints at some confidence and assertiveness. SHAPE an encounter for him to share this message with his imaginal boss, whose name is Ben.

How to Do Move 3 Shaping Encounters

Workouts for EFT Tango Move 3: SHAPE an Engaged Encounters

S Sharpen message (use reflection)
H Heighten (with repetition, proxy voice)
A Anticipate sharing and receiving (sometimes *seeding attachment*)
P Direct to **Present** (*slice thinner* if needed)
E Engage (redirect, refocus, catch bullets) if needed

Your Sharpening
Repeat the core message you are inviting Samir to share with his boss, owning his action tendency and his core emotional experience: _____
_____
_____

Emily's Sharpening
(Using proxy voice to sharpen.) So afraid you don't want me anymore – that I have let you down – afraid too of letting you down more – so I lie low and start to doubt myself – but I did make the right decision for my daughters and I'm getting tired and lonely in my hideout – I still have a lot to offer!

Your Heightening
Heighten with repetition of core phrases, with proxy voice: _____
_____
_____

Emily's Heightening
So afraid of letting Ben down, so I lie low, but – I made the right decision and I still have a lot to offer! (Emily uses his boss' name to heighten the experience by making it more personal and more real.)

Your Anticipating
Invite Samir to prepare to tell this clear message to an imaginal boss, noting how his boss looks as he prepares to share this with him, noticing how his body reacts as he anticipates sharing this with an imaginal boss. _____
_____
_____

Emily's Anticipating
Can you picture Ben just now as you prepare, in your imagination, to tell him, "I am afraid of your disappointment with me. I do lie low, but I do still have a lot to offer"? (Waits for Samir to respond.) What does he look like just now as you prepare to speak to him?

Your Directing Him to Present the message
Imagine Samir says, "He looks busy, kind of flat, cold, unapproachable." Begin by validating how challenging it is to speak to a cold, unapproachable boss, and persist with encouraging him to share the message (repeating it again): _____

Emily's Directing Him to Present the message

(Validating the challenge.) This is definitely challenging! Takes a lot of courage to tell this image of your cold, unapproachable boss how scary he is! This is very real, indeed. Very hard to imagine Ben would be open to hearing from you if you spoke to him! (Small seed of attachment) Can you tell him, "You are definitely frightening – so hard to approach – I live with this constant fear I've let you down and afraid of letting you down more" and if you can, tell him you know you made the right choice for your daughters and maybe add, that you know that you still have a lot to offer.

Your Engaging

Imagine Samir hesitates and says, "I can tell him I am scared I've let him down – but not the rest." To refocus him, you need to "slice the message thinner" into a manageable bite-size. Insert your refocusing with a thinner slice: _____

_____

_____

Emily's Engaging

(Refocusing and slicing thinner.) Good! Tell Ben how afraid you are that you have let him down and that for now it's just too difficult to tell him you do still have a lot to offer. Tell him that you just keep lying low and saying very little. Can you tell him that – still so afraid – not ready yet to let him know what you have to offer? Can you tell him that, please – "so afraid – certain I made the right decision – not able to tell you more yet"?

Your Strengths and Discoveries about Move 3

_____

_____

_____

Did you sharpen the message to share; heighten the emotionality in the message; safely help him anticipate the encounter; direct him to present the message while keeping the emotion alive; and refocus or engage where needed?

EFIT Tango Workout 8: Move 4 Processing an Engaged Encounter

How to Do Move 4 to Process Encounters

- Repeat the core of the message that was disclosed, using the client's words and non-verbals, such as eye contact, bodily movements, and voice change.
- Ask the discloser to describe their experience of sharing this message.
- Repeat the key verbal and non-verbal messages again and elicit the receiver's felt experience in receiving the message.

Read Samir's encounter below to his boss, aloud.

SAMIR: I am so afraid I let you down when I turned down that Middle East assignment. Terrified everyday. I lie low in fear you are disappointed with me… or have written me off because of my commitment to my daughters – or maybe it's because of the color of my skin. You look cold and scary. (Pauses, looks at therapist, then closes his eyes again as when he was speaking to his imaginal boss.) I just can't tell you yet that I still have a lot to offer – that I have ideas I'd like to share…

Your Move 4 Responses to Process the Encounter

1. Frame an evocative question to engage Samir in actively reflecting on his internal experience of having just disclosed to his imaginal boss (Create your style of asking how was it to share this message with his imaginal boss? Try including the key message he shared):

_____

2. Reflect, validate, heighten what you imagine Samir will answer – it may be a mix of fear and a glimmer of excitement at having actually had the courage to voice these words to an imaginal boss:

_____

3. Ask another evocative question to engage Samir in actively reflecting on how he experienced his imaginal boss to be reacting/looking/sounding:

_____

4. Elicit from Samir how it feels to get the response he imagines from his boss:

_____

Emily' Move 4 Responses to Process the Encounter

1. To evoke Samir's experience of having shared with his boss, Emily says: Samir, you just shared this important message with an imaginal Ben, how you are holding back, lying low in fear of his disappointment in you, and fearing you are being excluded because of your parenting responsibilities, or because of the color of your skin. And you even told him that it is too much right now to let him know that deep inside you do know you still have a lot to offer! What is happening inside for you as you share this and see his imaginal face?
2. Samir says it was very frightening and also a tiny bit exciting.
    To validate his present-moment experience of fear and a glimmer of excitement to be addressing him, Emily reflects and validates: Yes, quite frightening to step out of your lying-low pattern and to actually tell him of your fear, a fear so big, as you said, you can't tell him yet about knowing you have a lot to offer. Exciting too, that you actually spoke to him!
3. To elicit Samir's active reflection on how he experienced his imaginal boss, Emily asks, "How did Ben look, hearing this from you?"
    In response, Samir says, "I saw the slightest look of surprise on his face…something suggesting he may actually want to hear from me!"
4. To evoke, validate, and heighten his experience of this imaginal encounter, Emily responds, "It was so frightening to address him, and you actually saw a look of surprise on his face to hear from you – that said to you – 'just may-be he actually wants to hear from me!' How is that for you?"

Your Strengths and Discoveries about Move 4

_____

_____

Move 5. Emily frames a Move 5 summary of Samir's encounter with his boss – how he is feeling hopeful and encouraged to speak up more to him in real life. They linger to integrate this empowering experience of engaging with his unspoken confidence. Then Samir repeats what he said earlier, "I know I made the right choice in turning down that Middle East travel assignment, even if no one else agrees, because my daughters needed me, but now I barely know how to be with them!" They agree to return to this in a future session.

Move 5 Integration and Validation

- The goal of Move 5 is to integrate, validate, and summarize.
- It can be used in the midst of sessions and at the end of sessions.
- It can be used to summarize and heighten the corrective emotional experience of new moments of engaged contact.
- The summary, validation, and integration of Move 5 often feel like a celebration, focusing on positive affect and emotional balance.
- During Stage 1 Move 5 is useful to draw the contrast between the old cycle or pattern and the new moves they are taking or even the ways they are now able to stop the old pattern and talk about what they are doing and the fears driving them.
- In Stage 2 Move 5 includes highlighting the new moves and emerging emotions, and emerging shifts in views of self and other, *broaden-and-build* patterns, and growing attachment security.
- In Stage 3, Move 5 summarizes, validates, heightens, and consolidates the impacts of the new resilience and secure bonds and the picture of the future on this trajectory.

Micro-interventions for Move 5 include empathic tracking reflections of changes and change events, heightening, validating, and summarizing.

Move 1. Early in the next session, Emily joins with Samir in turning to the family relationships he identifies as being very important to him, reflecting with Move 1: Yes, you are very certain you make the right choice for your daughters! They are so important to you and you find it very troubling that you get stuck in knowing how to relate to them! Can we go back to what you were saying about how your daughters' laughter and excitement is a big trigger for your numbness and for the grief at losing your wife? Your daughters trigger so much that you have not been able to talk about all these years since Nahlah died. The more you notice your daughters, the more you see your wife in them and to stay away from your empty cavern of grief, you find yourself pulling away from them as well … lying low, saying very little, going numb, and having occasional, unpredictable outbursts.

EFIT Tango Workout 9: Move 2 Assembly in the Family Relational Context

Read Samir's words aloud.

SAMIR: As I've been saying, my daughters are important to me, but I don't know how to be with them! I hear their laughter; I see their enthusiasm, but I feel numb. Dalia's laughter sounds exactly like Nahlah and Amina (voice softens with a fragile tone), she looks more like her mother every day (grimace, pained face). Some days I catch a glance at her and for a split second I feel like Nahlah is back. I don't want to keep thinking of her! It's too much! I want to be a better parent (Deep sigh!) I'm proud of them – but I don't tell them. I barely feel it. (Pause.) I get irritable and just shout sometimes (sigh!) I am sorry – looks at the therapist. It's too much – (flat tone; expressionless face) I just need to carry on.

Your Inner Process and Attunement to form a Move 2 Assembly

1. Expressed elements of Samir's emotional experience? _____

_____

2. Hint of attachment panic or core, unexpressed emotion? _____

_____

3. Elements to expand with Move 2 evocative responses or questions? _____

_____

Your Move 2 Assembly, linking elements of emotion and forming a coherent story:

_____

_____

_____

Emily's Inner Process and Attunement to Form a Move 2 Assembly

1. Emily identifies the following elements of emotion Samir has expressed:

   Perceived threatening cue/trigger: Daughters' laughter and excitement; Amina looks more and more like her mother; Dalia's laughter sounds like Nahlah.
   Body: Voice breaks; soft, fragile voice, sighs, pauses, grimace, pained face, flat tone; expressionless face
   Meaning: Daughters are important; It's too much; doesn't know how to be with his daughters; wants to be a better parent.
   Action tendency: Tries to ignore feeling of how important daughters are to him; goes numb; tries to avoid thinking of his wife; just "carries on"; gets irritable, shouts.

2. Emily hears a hint of attachment panic in Samir's longings to be a good parent! She hears a hint of fear of failing. She also hears fear of loss, abandonment, and isolation, without his wife.

Emily's Move 2 Assembly
   She links these elements together in a Move 2 assembly to form a coherent story: I'd like to hear more about how your daughters' laughter and enthusiasm immediately bring memories of your wife alive. I hear that you love them so much, yet they trigger your deepest, unspeakable loss

and you go numb and do not interact with them as you would like to. Being reminded of Nahlah all feels like too much, so you just carry on, mostly numb, never daring to get close to them or to feel how much you miss your wife. Do I get it?

Your Strengths and Discoveries of Move 2 _____

_____

_____

After this assembly, Emily evokes more about how his daughter's laughter (cue) immediately triggers him to think of his wife and how he rapidly moves away (action tendency) from his daughters to also get away from thoughts of missing his wife. This trigger/immediate action tendency to avoid experiencing his grief is an important process to focus on.

She expands on Samir's action tendency to "just carry on," trying to be successful with work and parenting and deliberately staying away from how much he misses his wife. She validates that focusing on the daily responsibilities of parenting and carrying on at work makes sense, when he feels like he simply cannot dare to entertain thoughts of how much he misses his wife. She validates the pattern of avoidance as a strength. She also acknowledges the costs of this strategy and the huge amount of energy it takes. She helps Samir to deepen his ownership of his action tendency to move away from his daughters and from the cavern of emptiness, representing the feelings and thoughts of his beloved wife. To safely and respectfully broach the topic of his grief, she asks when, if ever, he and his daughters talk about their mother/his wife, Nahlah.

EFIT Tango Workout 10: Stage 1 Encounters to Own Action Tendency and Core Emotion

Encounters are typically shaped following the assembly of the *emotion-story* and the deepening of the core experience. Imagine there are multiple Stage 1 encounters shaped and processed with flows of Moves 2–4, where Samir owns his action tendency in the emotion regulation pattern of which he is both a participant and a prisoner. You have already shaped a Stage 1 encounter with his boss. Now, identify the other encounters you anticipate you would be shaping if he were your client. Stage 1 encounters function to make contact with a significant other or a part of self while owning and disclosing action tendencies. They also function to access or deepen the core emotions underlying automatic ways of coping.

Encounters and Their Function
Examples

With Nahlah, for Samir to acknowledge, he copes with missing her by trying not to think of her.
With Nahlah, for Samir to access the core anguish of missing her, that he ignores.
With daughters, with Amina, for example, to acknowledge how much she looks like her mother and reminds him of her mother, constantly. Or to acknowledge how he realizes he has been distancing to keep from feeling his grief.
With Dalia – to disclose how her laughter reminds him of her mother every time he hears it.
Now, it's your turn to identify who you would shape an encounter with and for what purpose. You can choose all the balloons (significant relationships.) To choose with whom to do an encounter, follow the emotion that is alive or the emotion which seems most difficult to access.

1. With whom:_____; Function: _____

_____

2. With whom: _____; Function: _____

_____

3. With whom: _____; Function: _____

_____

4. With whom:_____; Function: _____

_____

Encounters Emily Identifies and Their Function

1. With whom: Samir's imaginal daughters; <u>Function</u>: to make imaginal contact with them and acknowledge he is coping with his fear of feeling how much he misses their mother (core emotion) by distancing and sometimes lashing out at them (action tendencies) and to express the underlying pride he feels in them (core emotion).
2. With whom: An image of Nahlah; <u>Function</u>: to make imaginal contact with her – a huge step out of his typical pattern, to acknowledge he tries to avoid thinking of her (action tendency) to stay out of a bottomless cavern of grief that threatens to devour him (core fear).
3. With whom: His imaginal father; <u>Function</u>: to make imaginal contact with him and to acknowledge that he still protects him (action tendency) by saying he was a good father and ignoring the scars of shame and blame he carries from him (core emotion).
4. With whom: Between Samir's vulnerable, grieving, lonely self and his confident competent self that is emerging; <u>Function</u>: to acknowledge he is dismissing (action tendency) his core grief (core emotion) and to make contact with his disconnected grief-stricken self and his emotion process of disconnecting.

Your Strengths and Discoveries about Stage 1 Encounters

_____

_____

In Stage 1, multiple encounters are shaped and processed with flows of Moves 2–4, where Samir owns his action tendency in the emotion regulation pattern of which he is both a participant and a prisoner: to his boss, to his daughters, to Nahlah, his wife, to his now-deceased father whom he has protected from blame for his entire life and between the disregarded, grieving, hurting self and the emerging competent, coherent self, and with the therapist.

EFIT Tango Workout 11: A Block in Move 3 Encounter for Samir with His Daughters

Following the Move 2 assembly and deepening of Samir's emotional experience with his daughters, Emily shapes a simple Stage 1 encounter for Samir to speak to his imaginal daughters. Imagine Emily uses SHAPE (**S**harpen, **H**eighten, **A**nticipate), to help Samir encounter his daughters and to disclose a message they have formed together.

As she directs him to **P**resent the message to them, it unfolds as follows:

EMILY: *Can you picture Amina and Dalia, just now?* (Pause; Samir nods.) *Close your eyes if you'd like.* (He closes his eyes.) *And can you tell them, "I am proud of you – but so far I have not let myself feel that pride or tell you about being proud of you"?*

SAMIR: Amina and Dalia, I hear your laughter; I see your enthusiasm for your activities, your friends but I feel numb. I'm proud of you but – (Stops. Opens his eyes and looks at the therapist) I can't do this. I can't see them anymore.

This is a moment for the "**E**" in the acronym SHAPE – *to re-Engage*. Insert how you could re-focus Samir to re-engage him to continue this encounter. You may validate, repeat the cue, be transparent, or slice thinner.

Your Move 3 Response to Re-Engage Samir _____

_____

_____

Emily's Move 3 Response to Re-Engage Samir (Repeating cue to validate.) Seeing Amina whom you are so proud of, in your imagination, looking more and more like Nahlah, brings up so much emotion. You told them you are proud of them and suddenly you looked right at me and said, "I can't see them anymore." I am here, admiring your courage and hearing your struggle. (Therapist transparency and support.) Can you close your eyes even briefly just now and see Amina's beautiful face again? (Repeating cue to engage him in present-moment experience.) and can you tell her, "I am so proud of you, but when I see how much you look like your mother, I just go numb"? (Slicing it thinner, which makes it possible for Samir to re-engage in this disclosure.)

Your Strengths and Discoveries about re-engaging a client who gets blocked in doing an encounter

_____

_____

_____

EFIT Tango Workout 12: Move 4 to Process Encounter between Samir and His Daughters

Your Move 4 Engage Samir in reflecting on his internal experience of having just disclosed to his daughters, and specifically Amina, "I am so proud of you, but can't tell you yet - when I see how much you look like your mother, I just go numb."

_____

_____

_____

Emily's Move 4 to engage Samir in reflecting on what he has just disclosed What are you experiencing inside having just said to an image of your daughters that you are proud of them, but just can't let yourself feel it or tell them yet because you simply go numb when you see how much they remind you of Nahlah?

SAMIR: I feel it more now, the pride, just imagining telling them this, I can feel it is there. It is not too much now. Amina does look so much like Nahlah, but I am feeling just now that I am so proud of them both. I can feel it (Tears stream down his cheeks). These are good tears!

Follow with another evocative question.

Your Move 4, to evoke Samir's experience of his imaginal daughters' response

_____

_____

Emily's Move 4, to evoke Samir's experience of his imaginal daughters Your tears are flowing. How are you imagining your daughters are responding? How do they look, as you've told them you are proud of them, but you just can't tell them yet? That you just go numb with how much they remind you of their mother?
    Samir: They are smiling… just looking happy to hear from me! (More tears.)
    Follow this with evoking from Samir how it feels to take in their response and their smiles.

Your Move 4, to evoke Samir's experience as he absorbs his daughters smiling back

_____

Emily's Move 4, to evoke Samir's experience as he absorbs his daughters smiling back What is happening inside of you as you look in your daughters faces, especially Amina's, see their smiles and feel your pride in them?

SAMIR: Just huge relief! Like I am coming to life…and I want to tell them when I see them how proud of them I really am!

Your Strengths and Discoveries about Move 4 Processing Encounters

_____

_____

EFIT Tango Workout 13: Move 5 Integration

Consider the encounter you have shaped and processed with Moves 3 and 4 above. Create a Move 5 summary and validation, to integrate and savor the work you and Samir have just done.

Your Move 5 Summary and Validation

_____

_____

_____

Emily's Move 5 Summary and Validation. You've created an amazing experience here. Gradually you faced your beautiful daughter, Amina who looks so much like Nahlah, and Dalia whose laughter sounds like Nahlah, and as challenging as it was you faced your images of them and in telling them you are proud of them even though you rarely tell then, your feelings of pride began to come alive. It became safer to see and hear how much they remind you of Nahlah. Seeing their smiling faces responding to you gave you relief and stirred your sadness - what you call "good tears." Your connection with your daughters and your own grief for Nahlah are coming more safely alive, yes?

Your Strengths and Discoveries about Move 5 _____

_____

_____

Imagine that after this, there will be other Stage 1 Tango flow wherein Samir will be helped to own his typical imprisoning pattern of the more he distances from others and his own internal experience, the more others appear to distance from him and disregard or judge him and the more he feels disconnected from himself and others. As he says, "feeling like a wounded animal, caught in a cruel spin of holding back, avoiding, and experiencing others to be unsafe, excluding him and judging him." With Moves 1–4, the therapist helps him to identify this pattern and acknowledge it in encounters with significant others, in addition to his boss and daughters as seen above. He will process this pattern across relationships with his wife, his now-deceased father, and between his vulnerable, disregarded, lost self and his emerging competent, alive self.

EFIT Tango Workout 14: Move 1 Stabilizing with a New Relational Context (Stage 1 Continuing)

Read Samir's comments below aloud.

SAMIR: In many ways, my life is stabilizing. I am feeling better about myself, speaking up more in staff meetings at work, getting new journalistic assignments that appeal to me and are compatible with short travel that allows me to be with my daughters most overnights. My sense of excitement and competence are returning at work but going home after work (Long pause; throws up his hands; deep sigh before continuing.) – – – I am managing to interact a little more with my daughters, but home is still a huge threat of the empty cavern without Nahlah. I freeze less, but I still do go numb and hope the evening passes quickly.

Your Inner Process and Attunement
   Most poignant emotional impact communicated: _____
   Identify what triggers and threatens Samir: _____
   Identify what Samir does in response: _____
   Your bodily resonance with this pattern: _____

Your Tango Move 1. Use behavioral, nonjudgmental words. Indicate where you would pause in your response, to check if your words are accurately capturing Samir's experience. _____

_____

_____

_____

Emily's Inner Process and Attunement

The most poignant emotional impact: The sharp contrast between Samir's growing confidence and excitement at work and the persistent empty cavern of missing his wife which emerges when he returns home.

Triggers for Samir's empty cavern and freeze response: his daughters and their home without Nahlah.

What Samir does in response, to this lonely, missing place: Freezes, goes numb, and hopes his evenings pass quickly.

Bodily resonance: Emily resonates in her chest with a physical sensation of an empty cavern in sharp contrast to Samir's warmer, more included, and confident feelings at work.

Emily's Tango Move 1

So empty without your partner; parenting alone, yes? (Pause for him to confirm.) The sharp contrast seems to be growing: Amazing to be feeling included in your workplace again and engaging more openly with colleagues, even to be interacting a little more with your daughters, but that emptiness of how much you miss Nahlah whenever you return home is so very stark! The more competently you function at work and are included there, the more emptiness and longings for Nahlah arise when you return home, and you still freeze and go numb, yes?

Your Strengths and Discoveries _____

_____

_____

EFIT Tango Workout 15: Move 1 before Assembling Emotion, to Guide Samir into Stage 2

Continuing from Emily's Move 1 above, Samir responds as follows. Read his words aloud.

SAMIR: I am afraid now that Nahlah didn't really want to go to Palestine. I know we'd always talked of moving back to the refugee camp to expose our daughters to the life their grandparents came from – so they would know what it truly means to be Palestinian and would integrate Arabian values… but I am afraid it is my fault that she was killed while we were there. I think we made the wrong choice. (Pauses.) My father said it was a stupid idea to go to Palestine. Maybe he was right! Some days I feel I can't go on without her. I'm filled with doubts and uncertainties.

Your Inner Process and Attunement, while Forming a Move 1 Reflection

Most poignant emotional impact communicated _____

Identify what triggers and threatens Samir _____

Identify what Samir does in response _____

Your bodily resonance with this pattern. _____

Your Tango Move 1 _____

_____

_____

Emily's Inner Process and Attunement

Emily is most struck with Samir's questioning the decision to go to Palestine, doubting himself, regretting the decision, hearing his father's criticism, like many echoes in the empty cavern of his grief.

Key triggers for his grief: His daughters' laughter and happiness; the ways they resemble their mother; items in their home that remind him of Nahlah's absence.

She notes that what Samir immediately does (his action tendency) when he feels the empty cavern of missing Nahlah is to doubt if it was the right decision to have gone to Palestine; starts to blame himself; listens to his father's past criticism;

Emily's bodily resonance: Notices that the empty cavern in her chest now feels like a heavy weight!

Emily's Move 1 Tracking Reflection: The more your daughters and your home without Nahlah trigger your grief, the more you question what was your joint decision* to have gone to Palestine, fault yourself, and listen to your father's hurtful words, yes? (Samir nods). It's almost like questioning your decision to have gone to Palestine protects you from this empty cavern of missing Nahlah?

Samir whispers: It does... and I am remembering now that we definitely did make that decision together. It was a dream we shared!

* Note: Emily deliberately included "joint decision" in her reflection, to retain a focus on a facet of Samir's story that he typically mentions briefly and then quickly disregards in his self-protective pattern of questioning and judging himself. This strategy protects him from feeling his unalterable loss. As with most action tendencies, attachment strategies, and patterns, there is a protective function, and even a strength, but also a liability.

Your Strengths and Discoveries about Move 1 Reflection _____

_____

_____

EFIT Tango Workout 16: Move 2 Deepening into Stage 2

Imagine that Move 2 Assembly preceded this workout and we are now focusing on Move 2 deepening of Samir's core grief and loss. Assembly creates a coherent *emotion-story,* that opens the doors into deepening his core emotion.

Read Emily's Move 2 assembly of Samir's present-moment experience aloud to experience a felt sense of this *emotion-story.*

Emily's Move 2 Assembly, linking Samir's elements of emotion into a coherent emotion-story:

Amina's beautiful face, the sound of Dalia's laugh, every day, remind you more and more of Nahlah and of how much you miss her (repeating trigger). An empty cavern you identified in your chest and your stomach, deep inside, so much grief and sadness! When missing Nahlah is too hard to stay with, you slip into questioning and judging yourself (action tendency; meanings made). You hear your father's familiar, critical words, "What's wrong with you!" and you doubt yourself even more. When your body isn't frozen in numbness it is wracked with the pain of questioning, blaming, and regretting your decision, yes?

Samir confirms this assembly, "Exactly! Exactly!" (Big sigh, with his hand on his stomach.)

Your Inner Process and Attunement to Form Move 2 Deepening

1. Emotional handle that captures the assembled *emotion-story:* _____
2. Related somatic signals: _____
3. Your bodily resonance: _____

Your Tango Move 2 Deepening. Slowly and simply repeat the emotional handle, capturing the core *emotion-story* of his grief. Optionally, use proxy voice and/or focus on the bodily felt sense.

_____

_____

_____

Emily's Inner Process and Attunement to Form Move 2 Deepening

1. Emily resonates with the emotional handle of an *empty cavern,* how difficult it is for Samir to "stay there." Given how his protective action tendency automatically moves him into self-doubts and criticism to get away from this emptiness, in her empathic imagination, she senses it must be frightening to feel his grief.
2. She notices his deep sigh, his hand on his stomach, combined with this image of an empty cavern that captures his fear of the core grief that is so difficult to stay with.
3. She places her hand on her own stomach and feels a nauseous sensation.

Emily's Tango Move 2 Deepening: Can we stay with that empty cavern you identified in your chest and your stomach, deep inside, an empty cavern of so much grief and sadness at missing Nahlah? Frightening to feel that emptiness? (Adding a conjecture, based on her attunement.) Your hand is on your stomach, and you just took a deep sigh. Just notice what is happening there. Can you feel that empty cavern? (pause) Can you stay there and notice what comes up?

Your Strengths and Discoveries about Move 2 Deepening

_____

_____

A Spontaneous Encounter between Client and Therapist

In response to Emily's Move 2 deepening above, Samir takes a long pause. With his hand remaining on his belly, looking into Emily's eyes, in a slow voice, clearly emotionally engaging with each word he, says, "I think….I am afraid….to feel….that emptiness. Feels it will devour me…. safer not to stay there."

As part of the Move 2 assembly, Emily validates Samir's fear, in the context of his typical self-protective pattern.

EMILY: Yes, I hear you. It takes so much courage to notice that empty cavern when it feels it will devour you. It is safer to move into the old familiar pattern of blaming and doubting yourself for Nahlah's death! And you just felt it now, didn't you? (Samir nods). You felt the emptiness – life without Nahlah – and suddenly you looked at me and said, "I am afraid to feel that – it feels like the emptiness will devour me."

SAMIR: (Takes a tiny gasp, continuing to look at Emily.) Yes!

In this spontaneous encounter with Emily, Samir briefly feels his cavern of emptiness and loss, and in disclosing to Emily how afraid he is of that emptiness, deepens his awareness of how frightening it is to experience it, even momentarily.

EFIT Tango Workout 17: Move 4 to Process a Spontaneous Encounter between Client and Therapist

Keep the moment of the encounter alive and evoke the discloser's present-moment experience and share your present-moment experience as is relevant to the therapy process.

Samir suddenly looked directly at the therapist, saying, "I am afraid…to feel…that emptiness. Feels it will devour me."

Your Move 4 Responses to process and savor this encounter

1. Repeat the core of the message and ask Samir to describe his experience of sharing:

_____

_____

2. Repeat the message again and as the recipient of the disclosure, share how it felt to receive his message: _____

Emily's Move 4 Responses

1. (Repeating Samir's message, Emily invites Samir to tune into his experience):

With your hand, still on your belly, on that empty cavern, you just looked into my eyes and very courageously said, "I am afraid to feel this. I am terrified it will devour me." What is happening inside of you just now as you share with me how frightening it is to be doing what you are doing just now?

2. After Samir has time to process his inner experience of this new disclosure and to respond, Emily does the second part of Move 4. She discloses her experience of this encounter:

When you looked in my eyes, with your hand on that empty cavern of grief (places her hand on her own belly) and said, "I am afraid if I feel that emptiness, it will devour me," I could feel my heart swelling. I am so touched to see your bravery in letting me know how terrifying it is to feel your emptiness. And (adding, therapist transparency of the process) I want us to make it safe for you to pay attention to this cavern in a way that it will not devour you but will bring you closer to that loving connection you have with Nahlah.

To invite Samir to notice how he experiences her disclosure, she adds: How is it for you to hear me share this?

Your Strengths and Discoveries about Move 4 when Encounter is with Therapist

---

In response to Emily asking Samir how it is for him to hear her say, "*I want us to make it safe for you to pay attention to this cavern in a way that it will not devour you but will bring you closer to that loving connection you have with Nahlah,*" Samir replies, "I want to find that connection with her again….but… (voice rising, clearly irritated). But why did she have to step outside that day?! It was dangerous. There were protests. And we only had one more week left before returning to Canada?" (His face is pained).

Emily experiences Samir as though he is pleading with her to change reality and that makes total emotional sense to her. She is thrilled to experience Samir becoming more emotionally engaged and wants to join with him to maintain this deeper level of engagement. The most empathic response she can come up with is to validate his pain, matching his irritated tone, and linking his emotional pain to the explicit trigger: How painful! How unfair! Your final week there, and she was caught in the danger of a protest and did not survive!

Emily attunes with more Move 2 to coherently assemble and safely heighten and contain Samir's emerging edges of emotional experience. They explore his irritation and anger toward the protests and the dangers and poverty in the refugee camps. Much more personally, they explore what Samir calls his "shameful and irrational" anger at Nahlah for going outside that day. "I know it wasn't her fault, but I keep landing on this irritating sense of, "Why did you go outside! It was not safe!"

Emily shapes numerous Stage 2 restructuring encounters with Samir where together they begin to restructure his experience of his world and his sense of self and others. He has stabilized what he calls his cruel spin of avoiding and holding back emotions that feel too difficult and too alien or frightening to feel. He is moving from reactive self-blame and self-doubts to the core emotions in his unexplored grief. He discovers, jumbled in his grief, the triad of social pain (anger, sadness, and fear of loss) toward Nahlah.

Stage 2 Encounters to Disclose Core Emotion

Consider shaping Stage 2 engaged encounters with an imaginal Nahlah to help Samir disclose his core emotions that up until now have been too unfamiliar, frightening, and unacceptable to feel. Shaping these encounters could include, helping him to share: (a) his core anger at Nahlah for leaving the house during the dangerous situation where she was killed; (b) his grief, which emerges as he expresses the anger toward her and discovers depths of sadness and heartbreak that he had numbed along with his anger; and (c) his fears that he cannot go on without her; that he is lost without her and very much afraid of parenting without her.

These encounters will serve the functions of helping him to access, deepen, and disclose the core emotions and vulnerabilities underlying his automatic attempts to avoid thoughts and feelings of her. His repetitive emotion regulation patterns are undergoing shifts. Instead of going numb and blaming and doubting himself across his relationships and inside his own lonely, isolated, inner self, he is engaging in clear expressions of core emotions and sending clear signals of his anger, his sadness, and his fears.

In encounters with an imaginal Nahlah, he discloses his core anger and experiences that in his very real image of her loving face, she does not flinch. He senses that his imaginal Nahlah can hear him and accepts him fully. This opens Samir to find the words and the physical anguish of unexpressed core sadness and depths of fears of being totally lost and having no sense of who he is without her.

The remaining Stage 2 corrective emotional experience that can be shaped with engaged encounters is to support him to send a clear request to his imaginal Naleh, to secure the bond in his grief and to integrate this new experience. This "request encounter" is also known as a client's Step 7 – *a deliberate risk-filled and engaged reach to have attachment needs met.* From within these reprocessed core emotions of his grief – the anger, the sadness, and the fear, what *need* do you imagine Samir will access? What request can you imagine helping him to make of an imaginal Nahlah in an engaged encounter in Workout 18? Pause, to insert your conjecture here:

What need do you imagine Samir is likely to access from within his core attachment fear? ____
_____ (The answer from Samir will become clear as you continue.)

EFIT Tango Workout 18: Stage 2 Encounter with Nahlah to Send a Clear Request to Meet His Needs (aka Step 7)

Read Samir's statement below aloud.

SAMIR: Starting to explore this cavern that I have avoided; expressing things I felt were never to be spoken or even entertained in my mind, is opening new fields of possibilities for me. The empty cavern which used to threaten to destroy me is now filling in with huge, terrifying emotions, but it is becoming more terrifying to stay away from them. They are intense, but I can see them now. I can touch them. I am discovering from your responses and most of all from Nahlah's responses in our imaginary conversations, that my anger, my bottomless grief, my fears are acceptable – are normal. I feel her now in my heart. (He smiles and touches his heart.) She warms me. (Pauses.) I see her in the girls a lot, but now I have my own private connection with her too! (Smiles again with his hand remaining on his heart.) But I am still afraid of the emptiness … still afraid of how empty I am without her, especially as a dad, a family man, I am hollow, I have little to give.

SHAPE an encounter for him to access what he needs and to make a request to the imaginal Nahlah for this need, embedded in his core emotion.

Your Sharpening

Sharpen the core fear with RISSSSSC and initiate the search for his attachment need embedded in his core emotion. (Core emotion tells us what we need.) _____

Emily's Sharpening
Let's tune into this empty, hollow place, that is so afraid of being hollow, as a family man. You feel Nahlah, alive in your heart, warming your heart, but as a parent, you feel the empty, hollow cavern. Stay with the hollow, empty cavern to listen to what it needs from the imaginal Nahlah, in your heart. (Samir startles, looking pleasantly surprised.)

Your Heightening
Evoke and heighten the need embedded in his core fear: _____
_____
_____

Emily's Heightening
Listen to the empty cavern, so afraid (Switches to proxy voice.) I am hollow. I am nothing as a father without Nahlah. What does this hollow, empty, fear of nothingness need from your imaginal Nahlah?

Imagine Samir, continuing to look surprised, says, "I'd like her reassurance. To tell me I can do it. To remind me who she sees me to be. To tell me that I can be enough as a dad without her."

Your Anticipating
Help Samir to anticipate making the request for reassurance from Nahlah: _____
_____
_____

Emily's Anticipating
She is right there, in your heart listening to you. Can you close your eyes and picture her looking at you with all that tender love you have seen each time you've spoken with her in this way? How does she look just now as you prepare to ask her if she can give this reassurance you absolutely need to fill your empty cavern?

Imagine Samir responds, "She looks kind and warm – eager to do something for me!"

Your Directing to Present the Request
_____
_____
_____

Emily's Directing to Present the Request
Can you ask her? Can you ask her to give you this reassurance, to remind you that she trusts that you can be enough as a dad without her?

Imagine Samir says, after a long pause, "I want to. I want to ask her, I need to hear from her, but… but something keeps stopping me… He is interrupting me." (Long pause, without mentioning who is interrupting him.)

Your Engaging
When Samir appears to have exited somehow from his imaginal encounter and begins to talk about someone else, how might you provide a tracking reflection of what just happened, check in with him, replay the cue, and refocus him to (re)-engage him to complete the encounter? _____

_____
_____
_____

Emily's Engaging

You were picturing, Nahlah, feeling her warmth in your heart and trusting she actually wants to do something for you and were just about to ask her to reassure your empty, hollow fearful place that you are enough as a dad without her, and suddenly, you were interrupted by someone, yes?

Samir: All I could hear was my dad's voice, saying, "What's wrong with you!" There is plenty wrong with me, and I don't think I deserve to ask her this.

Emily: (Again directing Samir to present his request, uses reflection and validation.) Of course, if the voice from your harsh, rageful father has interrupted you it is very disruptive. We will take time to address your disruptive father later, but for now, let's ask him to wait, and we will stay with your warm image of Nahlah. Is that ok? (Maintaining focus to re-engage.)

Samir: (Looking shocked, then sighs in relief.) Ok. That's good.

Emily: I'd like you to make this important request of Nahlah. Can you let her know this is not easy – somehow your father's voice in your head keeps interrupting, but as you close your eyes, can you look again at her kind eyes, eager to do something for you, feel her warmth and let her hear your very important request? Can you ask to reassure you that she sees you as a good enough father?

Samir: Can you? Nahlah, do you believe in me? Can you tell me, do I have enough to give as a father without you? Am I more than a hollow shell as a father? Tell me you truly believe I can be more, much more to the girls than my father ever was to me. (He is shaking; beads of sweat appear on his forehead, and he sighs a huge sigh!)

You will be invited to reflect on your strengths and discoveries of Move 3 and 4 responses after you finish the next workout.

EFIT Tango Workout 19: Process Encounter with Nahlah

This may seem like a very different encounter to process, with the disruptive intrusion from his father's voice, but we will practice maintaining the focus on processing the engaged encounter of Samir's request to Nahlah. We will use the general Move 4 guidelines for processing this unique, highly risky encounter of making a clear *request* to have his attachment needs met.

Following Samir's clear request to Nahlah, immediately invite Samir to reflect on how he perceives Nahlah to respond to his request.

Your Move 4 to Evoke Samir's Present-Moment Experience (You may repeat the risk and the request he just made, as part of evoking and bringing his experience to life): _____

_____
_____

Emily's Move 4 to Evoke Samir's Present-Moment Experience

You just took this huge risk, even as you were interrupted rudely by your father's voice, you hung in and stayed focused on Nahlah's warmth and care and you took the risk to ask her to assure you that can be a good father to your girls, without her. How are you experiencing her response to you?

SAMIR: She's just there, loving me as always, assuring me over the top that I have always been the best dad they could want… reminding me that even when I've raised my voice it is very mild, and the girls totally trust me and love me and know that I am on their side. I just want to have more of these conversations with her. All these years I have never heard from her like this. It is amazing!

Your Strengths and Discoveries about Move 3 shaping this unique encounter of making a request to meet the need embedded in the core emotion and of your style of processing this request-encounter in Move 4 _____

_____

_____

SAMIR: That was incredible how we made my father wait while I was talking to Nahlah. First time in my life I could hear someone else's voice above his harsh criticism!

Now it is your turn – without Emily!

For the next two workouts – you are given prompts to follow, to guide you in creating your own EFT tango moves, without comparisons with Emily. Emily reappears for the final Move 5 workout.

EFIT Tango Workout 20: Moves 1–5 to Reprocess Samir's Relationship with His Abusive Father

Although Emily's responses are rarely given below for your comparisons, you can continue to *workout* and imagine your ongoing attunement with Samir through Moves 1–5 as you process his relationship with his abusive and unpredictably rageful father.

Before shaping the five moves described below, review the notes you have made where you have identified your strengths and any new facets you've seen in Emily's examples that you would like to integrate into your style. The slow, steady pace and empathic presence of an accessible, responsive, engaged therapist who is willing to walk with a client into the traumas they have only experienced in isolation provides tremendous resources for a client. This is how we harness the power of emotion and create change through interpersonal encounters.

Samir: I don't want to fault my father – I know he had a difficult life working for the Palestine Red Crescent Society. I know he suffered a lot and even after moving to Canada, I know he continued to suffer from things he saw and did and the time he was injured by a mob throwing stones at him.

Move 1 begins with validating how he always protects his father and disregards his own pain and shame from his father's abuse. The emotional handle for his experience is, "fighting a monster in my head, who is constantly calling me down and scoffing at me." With Move 1, you will validate the conflict Samir feels about discussing his father and the abusive damage that still rings in his head and in his body. For example, hearing, "What's the matter with you!" and during vulnerable moments, feeling tension and sharp pain firing up across his back where he still has scars from his father's belt. These are his cues – hearing his father's critical voice and feeling a burning pain in his back. His action tendencies are to protect his father, to say nothing, and to disregard his own shame and anger.

Your Move 1. Form a Tango Move 1 with behavioral, nonjudgmental words. In forming your Move 1, reflect and validate Samir's hesitancy to share any of his pain with his imaginal father and validate and heighten the pain and irritation he feels with regard to him.

You may indicate where you would pause in your response, to check if your words are accurately capturing Samir's experience. Formulate the link between trigger and response, and add the affect he is experiencing, if it is apparent: _____

_____

_____

_____

_____

Then, imagine Samir responds to your Move 1 by saying:

It is so hard to acknowledge how he hurt me, but I still feel that pain in my body and in my heart to-day. I know he suffered so much, but it was never ok that he beat me and belittled me like he did.

Begin to create a Move 2 assembly of his complex emotion of hurt toward his father for his abuse. In assembling the hurt you will access the complexity of assertive anger, sadness and grief, and fear, likely the fear of being rejected and hurt.

Your Move 2 Assembly. Insert your best attempt at linking elements of Samir's emotion: the trigger (for example, hearing his father's shaming voice), his bodily response (pain burning in his back), his mixed action tendencies (for example, wanting to shout back at him; wanting to slink away, saying nothing, even feeling sorry for his father's distress) and meaning-making (for example, views of self as deficient and unlovable, and of other as unpredictable and dangerous) together with his core anger, core sadness, and/or core fears.

_____

_____

Your Move 2 Deepening. Form your deepening response, by slowly and simply repeating an emotional handle, *(burning in my back; never ok that he beat me; never ok how he scoffed at me; heart-broken)* capturing the core, assembled *emotion-story* of his grief, assertive anger or fear. Optionally, use proxy voice and/or focus on the bodily felt sense. Here, you can imagine what other emotional handles may be emerging:

_____

_____

_____

Your Move 3, to SHAPE an Encounter

With Move 3, you can shape an encounter for him to disclose core emotion to his imaginal father, being careful to hold his father and not himself responsible for his father's hurtful actions toward his son. Collaborate with him to create safety for him, while shaping the encounter. For example, speaking to an imaginal other typically feels very real and risky for a client. To feel safe enough to speak to this image of his father, he may need to be certain that his father will not speak back or he may need to be assured that his father will listen and not crumble to the floor.

Ensuring Safety

Insert a statement and an evocative response or question that you could make to Samir to help identify what he needs to feel that he can face and speak to an image of his father: _____

_____

For example, he may create safety by telling his imaginal father that he will say his piece and he does not want to hear back from him.

SHAPE the Encounter

Sharpen his assertive anger toward his father. In the encounter, his anger may shift into grief and sadness for this ruptured relationship. He may focus on asserting the anguish of living with the unpredictability of a rageful, dangerous father (view of other). His core anger may begin with the fear of being deficient or living always in fear of hearing how defective he is, and never, ever having a safe father to count on. Choose an element from your imagined responses from Samir, that you will sharpen and support him to disclose in a safe engaged encounter with an image of his father. Using RISSSSSC, sharpen his core emotion: _____

_____

_____

Heighten with repetition, simply and slowly. If you are matching his emotional intensity with your voice, it may not be soft. You may use a firm, strong tone. Be specific in your words – specifically naming for what he has every right to be assertively angry at his father. (For example, "What you did was so wrong! You had no right to beat me like you did! This is how badly your unpredictable rages hurt me!") _____

_____

_____

Anticipate: Insert the words you will use to help him imagine his father, picturing how he looks, noticing how he feels in his own body as he prepares to address him. Resist taking him out of his experience by asking, "What would it be like to tell your father.?" _____

_____

_____

Present/Direct him to present the message to his imaginal father: _____

_____

_____

Engage. Imagine Samir exits or distracts from his imaginal encounter. How might you provide a tracking reflection of what just happened, check in with him, replay the cue, and refocus him to engage him to complete the encounter? _____

_____

_____

Your Move 4 Responses to Process the Encounter

Frame an evocative question to engage Samir in actively reflecting on his internal experience of having just disclosed to his imaginal father. (Try including the key message he shared): _____

_____

_____

Reflect, validate, heighten what you imagine Samir will answer. It may be a mix of fear and a glimmer of excitement at having actually had the courage to voice these words to an imaginal father: _____

_____

Follow with another evocative question to engage Samir in actively reflecting on how he experienced his imaginal father to be reacting/looking/sounding (if he wants to hear back from his father): _____

_____

Evoke from Samir how it feels to get the response he imagines from his father:

_____

_____

Now, determine if you want to shape more engaged encounters between the two of them. If so, take time after each Move 3 to process the encounter with another Move 4. _____

_____

_____

_____

Finally, use Move 3 and 4 to shape the pivotal encounter where he addresses his father with a request or an assertive limit. Having assembled and organized his emotional experience with his father, you will help him to access his need to request something from this image of his father or to assert permanent distance and make it clear he no longer wants a relationship with him.

_____

_____

_____

_____

_____

Your Move 5 Summary and Validation Form a validating summary of the work Samir did through these encounters:

_____

_____

_____

_____

_____

Your Strengths and Discoveries

Identify what stands out to you most from this experience of attuning with Samir with the five moves in relation to his abusive father. Take note of the courage it took on your part to walk into this difficult, painful territory so bravely, in safe, minute steps at the pace of Samir's readiness and within his window of tolerance: _____

_____

_____

_____

Identify any questions you may have to explore with your EFIT peer consultation colleagues. You may also consider watching an 11-hour EFIT training video series at steppingintoeft.com, that illustrates a client in several healing encounters with imaginal others who were abusive. The corrective emotional experiences for the client were a restructured view of self, and although they chose detachment from the abusive others, there was a shift in the working model of other by distinguishing those who cannot be trusted and were in the wrong, from others who can be trusted.

EFIT Tango Workout 21: Tango Moves for an Encounter between Two Parts of Self

As we saw earlier, in the midst of an encounter with Nahlah. Samir's imaginal father intruded. He interrupted Samir's warm encounter with Nahlah. You and Emily validated this disruptive moment and then, with a commitment to return to his father, retained the focus on his corrective emotional encounter with Nahlah. Imagine now, that in the midst of confronting his imaginal father to tell him how deeply he hurt him with his harsh words and his belt buckle, that Samir stopped, dropped his head, and turned to tell Emily that he sees his own sweet, innocent, sincere adolescent self. Emily invites him to follow the alive image of young Samir that has just appeared and to feel free to tell his imaginal father he needs to take a break but will return to tell him some very important things.

SAMIR: I am taking a break here, father. Young Samir has appeared and he needs my time.

Practice your growing capacity to shape encounters and create encounters between adult Samir and young Samir. The two parts of self are: (1) the sweet, innocent, adolescent self, vulnerable, disregarded, and in pain, in dialogue with (2) the present-day adult Samir whose sense of self is emerging as competent, loved, valued, and securely connected.

You can help him engage with each part: (1) the *disregarded, anguished self* which Samir has ignored – the part in pain, in shame, in grief, in love, full of emotions which have felt too difficult, foreign, or unacceptable for him to feel or articulate; (2) *the adult self* who is emerging with a sense of competence, valued and loved by others, and having a clear voice to reach and respond to others.

Your Tango Move 1. Form your Move 1 reflection of the present process with behavioral, nonjudgmental words. You may indicate where you would pause in your response, to check if your words are accurately capturing Samir's experience. Formulate the link between trigger and response:

_____

_____

_____

_____

_____

Your Move 1 attunement and reflection may be very different than the following example. It is just one possibility of tracking the present process between the two parts of Samir: Move 1 could involve tracking reflections of how it has been between these two parts of self, and how it seems to be shifting, as Samir is stabilizing and becoming more aware of his avoidant patterns. For example, "The more the competent, loved and loving Samir disregards the Samir in pain; the more disregarded Samir, in pain, slinks away in shame and says nothing. In contrast, the more the adult, competent, valued Samir pays attention to disregarded self's grief, anger, and fears, the more disregarded Samir is showing up and making himself heard."

Your Move 2 Assembly. Move 2 will involve assembling and deepening emotion in both the *disregarded self* and the *alive and valued self.* After a Move 1 that tracks the pattern between the two parts of self, you can assemble emotion with each part in turn. Before inserting your best attempt at linking elements of Samir's emotion, consider the elements of emotion for each part:

The trigger which evoked his awareness of the young, innocent, vulnerable, self in pain was the image of his abusive, rageful father.

A trigger that evoked his present-day adult Samir who is emerging as competent, loved, valued, and securely connected, was the image of his young self in pain;

Another trigger that evoked his new sense of being loved and cared for was the corrective emotional experience in dialogue with an imaginal Nahlah and requesting and receiving her assurance that he is a competent parent and he is still connected with her and is not alone.

The bodily response of his young, vulnerable self may have been when his head drops; he has described the burning sensation in his back from where he was beaten.

The bodily response of his present-day adult Samir may be the warm smile that crosses his face when his young self appears in his imagination.

The meanings made by his young self may be that, "I am somehow defective, given how harshly my father treats me; my father cannot help himself/he is in pain; he is unpredictable and dangerous; no one sees my pain."

The meanings made by his adult, growing-in-confidence-and-connection may be, "Young Samir is alone and hurting; he is innocent and he needs my love and protection; I am beginning to have a voice and have some power and am feeling Nahlah's love again and I have love to give my young self."

The action tendencies of his young self: Remains quiet, hangs head, slinks away, and disappears.

The action tendencies of his adult self: Standing up for young Samir; having a voice to tell father to wait while he attends to young Samir; regarding the young Samir with compassion.

Insert your choice of a Move 2 to assemble and link Samir's elements of emotion for each part of self – the adult and the vulnerable adolescent:

You could begin with the trigger for young Samir: You see this young, innocent, Samir, in so much pain, yet bravely smiling, doing all he can to disregard how difficult it is for him. (Continue, adding meanings, action tendencies, etc.): _____

_____

_____

Now link the elements of emotion for the adult Samir. You could again, begin with the trigger: The minute the young Samir appeared in your imagination, a compassionate smile crossed your face… (Continue, adding meanings, and action tendency.)

_____

Add your sense of the core emotion for each part (core anger, sadness, and/or core fears):

_____

Your Tango Move 2 Deepening. Form your deepening response, by slowly and simply repeating an emotional handle, capture the core, assembled *emotion-story* of Samir's disregarded, young self in pain and of his present-day adult self who is moving out of avoidance and disregard for his pain into recognizing what he is experiencing.

Optionally, use proxy voice and/or begin with the bodily sensations you imagine arising for Samir or showing up in his bodily movements. (For example, he has described the burning sensation in his back; he has a smile in recognition of his young innocence.) Here, you can imagine what other emotional handles may be emerging.

Deepen the emotional experience of young Samir: _____

_____

_____

Deepen the emotional experience of adult Samir: _____

_____

_____

Your Tango Move 3

With Move 3 you can shape engaged encounters between the anguished, disregarded adolescent self and the newly alive, loved, and loving adult self. Change events shaped through these encounters will be corrective emotional experiences of (1) an engagement change event where the previously disregarded, anguished self sends clear messages of fear and pain and asks to be loved and accepted, and (2) a softening change event of messages of love and acceptance from the alive, competent, loving self to the self in need of comfort and love.

What message may you shape for the young self to share with the adult self?

_____

_____

_____

What message may you shape for the adult self to send to the young self?

_____

_____

_____

Your Tango Move 4

With Move 4 process the impact of each encounter between two parts of Samir, validating and integrating. How is it to share? How is it to hear? Bullets may need to be caught (if self-criticism or denigration emerges) as you process the encounters.

_____

_____

_____

_____

_____

Imagine, after Move 4, that Samir adds:

I see myself, down on my knees, talking with young Samir, just a few years younger than Dalia. He is so bewildered and so sad. I tell him how perfect he is and how I wish I could take him out of this dangerous home. We lock eyes. I tell him I am so sorry I cannot save him from all the pain in his house and all the bad things that will happen, but that I will always be with him to protect his heart.

Your Tango Move 5

With Move 5, summarize, validate, and integrate the restructuring through these corrective emotional experiences.

_____

_____

_____

_____

_____

EFIT Tango Workout 22: Move 5 to Summarize and Integrate Samir's Changes across Relationships and Contexts

Below, insert your best summary to integrate, highlight, and savor Samir's corrective emotional experiences across relationship contexts and how these changes are all coming together in a new way of regulating emotion. You may include Stage 2 corrective emotional experiences at his workplace, with his daughters, in his relationship with his deceased wife, Nahlah, and his imaginal father. You may also include how the changes created through his interpersonal dialogues are expanding into his internal emotional regulation patterns where his secure connections with others, especially his close colleagues, his deceased wife, and his daughters are enlarging his internal world and expanding his relationship with self.

Of course, you will be using your imagination to comment on his corrective emotional experiences, coalescing in new *broaden-and-build* cycles: These cycles foster positive working models of self and other, secure ways of co-regulating emotion, and a capacity to internalize others' comfort so that he can access comfort internally as well. You may also paint a picture of his future, given the trajectory of his changes and the *broaden-and-build pattern.*

Your Move 5 Summary of Samir's Stage 2 Corrective Emotional Experiences

_____

_____

_____

_____

_____

_____

_____

Emily's Move 5 Summary of Samir's Stage 2 Corrective Emotional Experiences

Having confronted your deepest fears and anguish, you have reshaped your relationships with your daughters where you are now able to enjoy and engage with them. You are able to talk freely with them about their mother and sense how alive Nahlah is in their smiles and their laughter. You are now safe to feel the ache in your heart for Nahlah and also the joy of your connection with her. Your work relationships are nourishing your sense of creativity and confidence. You are speaking up more at work with your boss, just as you have with your imaginal father and feeling a new confidence and motivation to reach out and make new friends, and you are beginning to consider readiness for dating again. And that new connection you are fostering with the young Samir, when your confidence gets shaky seems like a powerful way you are building on the love you feel from and to others. I hear you saying, "That shaky little self, inside, is a good core, and I want to listen to him" yes?

Your Final Strengths and Discoveries _____

_____

Part 3

Self-of-the-Therapist Workouts

Table of Contents

There are many resources inherent in the EFT model that you can draw on for personal support as you blaze trails with your clients. Part 3 provides you with three types of workouts to help the EFT therapist foster their own balance and growth with the tools of EFT. All workouts in this book can be enhanced by joining with a colleague for practice and validation. You will learn from one another and will receive validation for your unique style of utilizing the same micro-skills and moves. The workouts in Part 3 are no exception. Working with a partner or small group is sure to enrich your self-of-therapist explorations.

First, in Part 3.1, is a detailed guide of journaling workouts with the moves of the EFT Tango to shape personal Stage 1 and Stage 2 change. This has frequently been used in EFIT training. Participants find journaling one evening prepares them to participate in a tango exercise with an engaged responder the next day. You can use this workout simply as a private journal activity, yet your experience will no doubt be significantly enhanced if it becomes an interpersonal one with a trusted, engaged responder.

Second, in Part 3.2, are reflection workouts to explore your level of comfort, and your barriers and strengths in the processes of lingering with, following, and deepening emotion. The explorations that can be engendered from these reflection questions are sure to take you into a very rich exploration with a colleague. Finally, in Part 3.3, to guide the reader-practitioner in continual pursuit of growth and hopefulness, is a goal-setting workout accompanied by a series of antidotes and resources inherent in the EFT model. You are invited to use this workout for goal setting along your journey of learning EFT. It is something to return to over and over again as puzzles and complexities arise with your clients.

PART 3.1: JOURNALING WORKOUTS WITH THE MOVES OF THE EFT TANGO

Journaling Workouts with the Moves of the EFT Tango in Stage 1 Stabilization

1. **Move 1 – Reflect Present Process**: Begin with journaling about a negative cycle in your life with someone important to you.

   a. Can you identify a vulnerable, core emotion that you tend to automatically bypass and instead become reactive in order to protect yourself? The most vulnerable emotions are likely to be some form of attachment danger such as fear of abandonment, rejection, or annihilation.

DOI: 10.4324/9781003242666-3

b. If you are unaware of bypassing a vulnerable emotion (because we do not like to dwell on them), simply choose to describe a familiar negative pattern – and jot down your reactive self-protective moves. For example, you may be inclined to ignore self and other, or to complain loudly about others, or to berate yourself.

2. **Move 2 – Assemble and Deepen Emotion**: Now describe the cascade of reactive responses that rapidly replace this moment of vulnerability (bodily arousal, meanings, reactive affect, and action impulses). Here are some evocative questions to guide your journaling:

    a. "Can you identify a danger cue or interpersonal trigger that you perceive as threatening (what you see or hear that begins this rapid cascade of unfolding elements of emotion)?
    b. What bodily sensations do you experience? What meaning do you make of this trigger and what is your automatic impulse to action?"
    c. Write out an empathic reflection to your answers to each evocative question above. Responding with empathy to yourself can deepen your emotional experience and enhance your self-reflective capacity to linger in emotional depth.
    d. Identify one emotion that comes up when you say, "When I see/hear (the interpersonal trigger) _____, I immediately do/feeling like doing (your action impulse) _____." Jot down how you feel about having formulated this. Linger for a few moments with the experience of that core, vulnerable emotion. You are not trying to create change. You are simply disclosing *what is* and how you are participating in your reality.

3. **Move 3 – Shape an Encounter**: Close your eyes and imagine a relevant other with whom to share this distilled message. This other could be an attachment figure or it could be a part of you (a younger or vulnerable image of self). See the other in your imagination – where they are, what they look like – and write out the most important part of this coherent message, as if you were disclosing it to this relevant other.

4. **Move 4 – Process the Impact of the Encounter**: Write down your experience of this imagined encounter. Describe how it was for you and how you imagine the other to be responding to this encounter. In your journaling, you may choose to write several exchanges back and forth between.

5. **Move 5 – Celebrate and Integrate**: Complete your journal entry by summarizing and celebrating the courage it took to have these imagined dialogues and how it is impacting you in this moment.

Journaling Workouts with the Moves of the EFT Tango in Stage 2 Restructuring

Move 1: Reflect Present Process

Recall a pattern you accessed in the previous self-reflection exercise. If you were unable to access a core fear, or cannot access it in this moment, scan your present-moment experience for something of importance to explore. Scan your body, your thoughts, and your impulses to action. Choose a difficult internal or interpersonal interaction, a bodily felt sense, a troubling perception, a pressing action impulse, or your core fear if it is within your awareness. Pay attention and prepare to linger with this and explore it. Jot down the key elements in your awareness, being sure to include the cue and your action tendency. What is it about that trigger (cue) that suggests, "Danger! Be on the alert!"?

Move 2: Assemble and Deepen Emotion

Reread what you have just written about this common cascade of personal emotion and describe your physiological experience as you review it. Linger in that bodily felt sense. Attune to the links between the cue, your action impulse, and the meanings you make of it. The process of linking these elements of emotion may be like opening doorways into experiencing your core attachment fear, underlying this process.

Write out a validation for the links of your own emotional experience (trigger/perception of danger, bodily response, meaning made, and action tendency) and do your best to name the core, underlying fear. Linger with this core emotion, even if it is best described as *numbness* or *nothingness*. Honor the feeling – welcome it with kindness and curiosity.

Describe in your journaling, an *emotional handle* – a poignant image, phrase, or bodily sensation that emerges. Linger with the emotional handle. Notice, if you can, what it is like to linger in core emotion without pushing it down or ramping it up. What is happening for you as you stay with that experience? How do you give yourself permission to linger there? Pay attention to any message, or meanings, or shifts you experience from within that emotion as you write more about your experience.

It is important to keep a *working distance* from this emotion, so that you do not lose your capacity to reflect and engage with the emotion. If you become flooded or overwhelmed, step back, name what is happening, and connect with a safe other or *imagined safe other* for support. Seek the support you need in order to return to the core emotion from a place of safety and emotional balance.

Describe any messages or shifts that are emerging. Listen for embedded needs, messages, new views of self or other, and longings or impulses to action that may emerge. Be simple: Anger calls for limits or to be heard; fear calls for protection; sadness calls for comfort; shame calls for disappearing.

Move 3: Shape an Engaged Encounter

a. *Choose the relevant other:* Linger again in your bodily felt sense of your core attachment fear or vulnerability, fully tasting, sensing, and experiencing it. Write the key distilled message that captures the core of this underlying emotion or attachment fear that you identified in your earlier journaling. Sharpen and heighten the message.

   If you are not already imagining a relevant other with whom to share this message, pause to consider who comes to mind as a relevant other with whom you need to disclose that vulnerability or fear? Is the core emotion an attachment fear? Perhaps it is an as-yet-unexpressed core anger and your message is an assertive message of core anger. Take time to linger and find the words.

   Ask yourself, with whom is this emotion most alive? or most blocked? or which attachment figure may be the best resource in this moment?

   You might ask yourself, "Whom do I need to hear this message – to truly hear me and be impacted by my truth?" Or, "Who is a trustworthy attachment figure I can call on to support me in this difficult moment?"

   You may discover it is a part of yourself you wish to address – a younger, more vulnerable part, or a compassionate adult part, or an estranged, unresponsive, or critical part.

b. *Anticipate making contact with this relevant other or part of self.* Begin describing in your journal, this relevant other, or this distinct part of self. Describe their physical features and describe what happens inside of you as you picture them about to receive this message from you.

c. *Express a clear message.* Take the risk of stepping forward, in your imagination to express your key message to the other. Write in your journal, as you imagine yourself expressing it out loud to the relevant other or to a part of yourself.

Move 4: Process the Experience

Pause and absorb how it feels to have put your clear request out to the other person (e.g., intense relief, deep comfort, dissipation of fear, or increased intensity of fear). Take in the enormity of the risk you have taken to make this disclosure.

Now begin to write again and this time write down how you imagine the other is responding to you. Write your imagined response as if you were writing from the other person/from the other part of yourself.

Pay attention to your inner experience as you imagine receiving this response. Feel free to choose to write several exchanges back and forth between *the two of you,* responding and receiving. (Several Moves 3 and 4, in dialogue.)

Option: *Make a reach from engaged emotion to make a request of the other.* (Another Move 3.) Check inside whether there is a yet-unexpressed need, embedded in that bodily felt vulnerable emotion – something you can risk requesting of the other. If the exchange was between a vulnerable part of self and a stronger, more stable part of self, the request may be from the vulnerable part to the stronger part. Write until your vulnerable need can be stated as a clear request. This is to be an actual request for something your core fear tells you that you need from the other to meet your attachment longing or need. Write out a specific "ask." Take the risk to write this request as if you were actually writing to this person or part of self that you are picturing as an actual person, and whose presence you can imagine. Ask for the core longing and need embedded in your fear. For example, "Can you reassure me I am valuable in your eyes? Can you assure me there is something specific about me that you like, that you treasure?" Write your imagined response from the other, as well, as if you were writing back from that imagined other or part of self. Describe how it is to receive this response to your request.

Move 5: Summarize, Integrate, and Celebrate the Experience

Give yourself time to write freely now to summarize what you have just done and to integrate and celebrate the corrective emotional experience you have created.

Note of assurance: If you have difficulty sending clear messages to an *imagined other* or cannot imagine *the other* responding favorably, simply observe and make a gentle note about what got in the way. As in therapy, the goal in personal reflection exercises is to stay with the process, validate it, *knowing that in an attachment frame, everything makes sense*, and blocked emotions always need to be respected, acknowledged, and further expanded and processed. Common blocks that people identify include, having difficulty keeping focused, getting flooded because the risk seems too great, flipping into reactive anger and blaming and turning away from the one they were approaching, and wanting to run from an experience that feels too risky or too hard to trust.

PART 3.2: REFLECTION WORKOUTS ON *LINGERING WITH* AND *FOLLOWING EMOTION*

Following the attachment map toward change in EFT means following the client's emotional experience. To do effective EFT, many therapists find they need to explore their comfort with and assumptions about emotion. Emotion is a verb. It is an active process that cannot be contained in one word. And many clients do not have a feeling word to describe their experience. One of an EFT therapist's greatest tools is understanding how emotion is an active trigger-perception-sensation-meaning-action process. Thus, whether working with a client who has little access to their emotional experience or a with client who is flooded with emotional reactivity or unrestrained verbal expressions, an EFT therapist has the tools to reflect present-moment process with unconditional acceptance and no need to move a client beyond where they are, and then assembling, beginning with whatever element of emotion is within the client's awareness.

Read the following questions to take note of your own comfort and conceptual awareness about lingering with and following emotion. For more detail on emotion, refer to Chapters 6 and 12 in *Stepping into Emotionally Focused Therapy.*

Do you prefer to try to get someone to *see it differently* or to *understand*, so their emotional experience is less distressing for them?

Are you confident with the power of simple reflection, specific, coherent validation, and your accepting presence to help a client regulate overwhelming emotion?

Are you challenged with assembling the elements of emotion?

Do you recognize in the moment that a client who does not use *feeling words* or experience any bodily sensations may be having an intense experience? Do you remember that emotion is more than a feeling word? It is an active trigger-perception-sensation-meaning-action process and clients are not likely aware of all these elements. Do you recall, in the moment that, "What that (trigger) says to you" and "What you typically do," or "What you feel like doing" are all elements of emotion and important handles to begin exploration?

Do you stop assembling or expanding an emotion once you have named it, assuming you and your clients fully grasp their experience?

Do you trust the process of engaging with *what is* – versus trying to change or fix?

When reactive emotion emerges, do you assemble it so as to validate specifically how it makes sense in that particular context, or do you *conjecture your way past it*? It can be very tempting to want to avoid reactive emotions and conjecture at an emotion that is more comfortable for the therapist or in EFCT, for the partner.

When core, unformulated anger emerges, do you assemble and deepen or sidestep it?

What other dynamics emerge as challenges or blocks for you in staying with and following present-moment emotion?

The most beneficial way to use this *reflection workout* would likely be to find a colleague to discuss each of your responses to these questions. Together you could identify and share your strengths in working with emotion and where you are challenged. You could collaborate on committing to a specific goal to increase your comfort, understanding, and capacity to savor, linger with, and deepen emotion or to regulate where needed and to follow the process of emotion into increasingly tolerable depths.

PART 3.3: WORKOUT TO SET LEARNING GOALS: ANTIDOTES TO COMMON EFT CHALLENGES

The following resources from within the EFT model are presented as antidotes to common challenges faced by therapists learning EFT. The EFT resource or intervention is presented in the first part of the sentence, followed by the common challenge.

You are encouraged to use this list to identify one or two learning goals for yourself. Focus on mastering your chosen goal(s) until you develop confidence and comfort with it. Return often to the list to set up your next goal, recognizing that within the model are extensive resources for challenges and confusion, faced by countless therapists.

1. Interrupt to find focus, rather than allow the client to continue unfocused and at a distance from their emotional experience. (Levels 1–3 on the Experiencing Scale.)
2. Reflect longings, collaborate with the client to set concrete, realistic, and positive goals, to be focused, rather than experience that you and/or the clients are directionless or overwhelmed.
3. Normalize distress: Assemble elements of emotion to identify the pattern as the problem – rather than getting caught up in the client's distress.
4. Show empathic curiosity to racial, gender, and social-contextual differences, rather than assume you understand, before you have listened deeply.
5. Enter the client's experience by starting with the element of emotion to which they have access. Use that to evoke other elements, rather than getting stuck in a search for *feeling words* or a bodily felt sense.
6. Validate reactive emotion and action tendencies, in the context of the client's specific elements of emotion (meanings, triggers, bodily sensations, consequences, and social context).
7. Find focus with reflection, rather than enthusiastically encouraging all emotional expression.
8. Stay within the client's *window of tolerance* – assemble *process of emotion*, validate reactive emotion, and heighten core emotion, rather than be flooded by incoherent emotionality or lost in disconnection.
9. Walk directly into pain with the client, rather than stay with content and problem-solving.
10. Assemble present-moment experience, rather than explore "why" (explanations/insights).
11. Slow down to stay with emerging edges of emotional experience (deepening to Levels 4–7 on the Experiencing Scale), rather than rushing on or making big conjectures.
12. Return to key emotional handles to re-engage when the client exits or when you lose focus.
13. Flow with Tango Moves 2, 3, and 4, to discover in collaboration with the client, the relevant other with whom to shape an encounter, rather than fearing you must choose the *correct encounter*.
14. Validate non-affiliation and authenticity during imagined encounters, rather than *side step it for something soft*.
15. Engage the resources in core anger and assertiveness, rather than dismiss all anger in favor of *softer emotion*.

References

Bowlby, J. (1988). *A secure base*. Basic Books.

Brubacher, L. L. (2018). *Stepping into emotionally focused couple therapy: Key ingredients of change*. Routledge.

Brubacher, L. L., & Wiebe, S. A. (2019). Process-research to practice in emotionally focused couple therapy: A map for reflective practice. *Journal of Family Psychotherapy*, *30*(4), 292–313. https://doi.org/10.1080/08975353.2019.1679608

Conrad, C. A. (2015). The evolution of an emotionally focused therapist: A mixed-methods research study. EFT Community News, 16, 6–7.

David, S. (2016). *Emotional agility: Get unstuck, embrace change, and thrive in work and life*. Avery.

Greenman, P. S., & Johnson, S. M. (2013). Process research on emotionally focused therapy (EFT) for couples: Linking theory to practice. Family Process, 52, 46–61. https://doi.org/10.1111/famp.12015

Johnson, S. M. (2004). *The practice of emotionally focused couple therapy: Creating connection* (2nd ed.). Brunner-Routledge.

Johnson, S. M. (2009). Attachment theory and emotionally focused therapy for individuals and couples. In J. H. Obegi & E. Berant (Eds.), *Attachment theory and research in clinical work with adults* (pp. 410–433). Guilford Press.

Johnson, S. M. (2019). *Attachment theory in practice: Emotionally focused therapy with individuals, couples, and families*. Guilford Press.

Johnson, S. M. (2020). *The practice of emotionally focused couple therapy: Creating Connection* (3rd ed.). Routledge.

Johnson, S. M., & Brubacher, L. (2016). Emotionally focused couples therapy: Empiricism and art. In T. Sexton & J. Lebow (Eds.), *Handbook of family therapy* (pp. 326–348). Brunner/Routledge.

Klein, M. H., Mathieu, P. L., Gendlin, E. T., & Kiesler, D. J. (1969). The experiencing scale. A research and training manual (Vol. I). Wisconsin Psychiatric Institute.

Klein, M. H., Mathieu-Coughlan, P., & Kiesler, D. J. (1986). The experiencing scales. In L. S. Greenberg & W. M. Pinsof (Eds.), *The psychotherapeutic process: A research handbook* (pp. 21–71). Guilford.

Koren, R., Woolley, S. R., Danis, I., & Török, S. (2022). Training therapists in emotionally focused therapy: A longitudinal and cross-sectional analysis. *Journal of Marital and Family Therapy*, *48*, 709–725. https://doi.org/10.1111/jmft.12495

Martin, D. (2016). *Counseling and therapy skills* (4th ed.). Waveland Press.

Mikulincer, M., & Shaver, P. R. (2023). *Attachment theory applied: Fostering personal Growth through healthy relationships*. Guilford.

Pascual-Leone, A., & Yeryomenko, N. (2017). The client "experiencing" scale as a predictor of treatment outcomes: A meta-analysis on psychotherapy process. *Psychotherapy Research*, *27*(6), 653–665. https://doi.org/10.1080/10503307.2016.1152409

Rice, L. N. (1974). The evocative function of the therapist. In D. A. Wexler & L. N. Rice (Eds.), *Innovations in client-centered therapy* (pp. 289–311). Wiley.

Rodríguez-González, M., Schweer-Collins, M., Greenman, P. G., Lafontaine, M.-F., Fatás, M., & Sandberg, J. G. (2020). Short-term and long-term effects of training in EFT: A multi-national study in Spanish-speaking countries. *Journal of Marital and Family Therapy*, *46*(2), 304–320.

Rousmaniere, T. (2019). *Mastering the inner skills of psychotherapy: A deliberate practice manual*. Gold Lantern Books.

Rousmaniere, T., Goodyear, R. K., Miller, S. D., & Wampold, B. E. (2017). *The cycle of excellence: Using deliberate practice to improve supervision and training*. Wiley Blackwell.

Sandberg, J. G., & Knestel, A. (2011). The experience of learning emotionally focused couples therapy. Journal of Marital and Family Therapy, 37(4), 398–410.

Skovholt, T. M. (2012). *Becoming a therapist: On the path to mastery*. John Wiley & Sons.

Watkins, C. E., Jr. (2012). On demoralization, therapist identity development, and persuasion and healing in psychotherapy supervision. *Journal of Psychotherapy Integration, 22*(3), 187–205. https://doi.org/10.1037/a0028870

Index